C000254578

PROTECTING CHILDREN AND YOUNG PEOPLE

Child Protection and Disability:
Methodological and practical challenges for research

PROTECTING CHILDREN AND YOUNG PEOPLE

SERIES EDITORS

JOHN DEVANEY
School of Sociology, Social Policy and Social Work, Queen's University Belfast

and JULIE TAYLOR
School of Health and Population Sciences, University of Birmingham

and SHARON VINCENT
Social Work and Communities, Northumbria University, Newcastle

Child Protection and Disability:
Methodological and practical challenges for research

Deborah Fry
Lecturer in Child Protection, Moray House School of Education, University of Edinburgh

Patricia Lannen
Program Director Child Protection, UBS Optimus Foundation, Zurich

Jennifer Vanderminden
Assistant Professor of Sociology, University of North Carolina, Wilmington

Audrey Cameron
Associate Tutor (Deaf Education), Moray House School of Education, University of Edinburgh

and

Tabitha Casey
Project Manager for the Safe Inclusive Schools Network, Moray House School of Education, University of Edinburgh

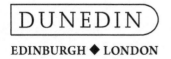

EDINBURGH ◆ LONDON

First published in 2017 by Dunedin Academic Press Ltd.
Head Office: Hudson House, 8 Albany Street, Edinburgh EH1 3QB
London Office: 352 Cromwell Tower, Barbican, London EC2Y 8NB

ISBN: 978–1–78046–050–5 (Paperback)
            978–1–78046–575–3 (ePub)
            978–1–78046–576–0 (Kindle edition)
ISSN: 1756–0691

British Library Cataloguing in Publication data
A catalogue record for this book is available at the British Library

Typeset by Makar Publishing Production, Edinburgh, Scotland
Printed in Great Britain by CPI Antony Rowe

CONTENTS

ACKNOWLEDGEMENTS

The authors would like to thank Dr Margit Averdijk, Dr Linda Bartolomei, Dr Ko Ling Chan, Professor Manuel Eisner, Dr Anita Franklin, Sofia Hedjam, Dr Berni Kelly, Dr Hannah Kuper, Dr Nambusi Kyegombe, Dipak Naker, Dr Denis Ribeaud, Sarah Rizk and Dr Desmond Runyan for their contributions to the case studies featured in this book. The authors would also like to thank Nick Drey, Caroline Bryson, Steven Webster and Matt Barnard from the National Society for the Prevention of Cruelty to Children (NSPCC) for their contribution of the consent guidelines table (Figure A.1) and Dr Susanna Niehaus for her contributions on social perceptions. The authors are immensely grateful to all contributors for their efforts to advance the state of knowledge around ethical research involving children with disabilities and commend their dedicated work.

GLOSSARY OF ABBREVIATIONS

ADHD	attention deficit hyperactivity disorder
ANOVA	analysis of variance
ASL	American Sign Language
BSL	British Sign Language
CP MERG	Child Protection Monitoring and Evaluation Reference Group
CPS	Child Protection Services
CRPD	Convention on the Rights of Persons with Disabilities
CSE	child sexual exploitation
DDTCP	Deaf and Disabled Children Talking about Child Protection
DSM	*Diagnostic and Statistical Manual of Mental Disorders*
ERIC	Ethical Research Involving Children
IRB	Institutional Review Boards
ISPCAN	International Society for the Prevention of Child Abuse and Neglect
JVQ	Juvenile Victimization Questionnaire
LMIC	low- and middle-income countries
LONGSCAN	Longitudinal Studies Consortium on Child Abuse and Neglect
LSF	Langue des Signes Française
MDGs	Millennium Development Goals
NatSCEV	National Survey of Children's Exposure to Violence
NCANDS	National Child Abuse and Neglect Data System
NCVS	National Crime Victimization Survey
NIS	National Incidence Study
NSCAW	National Survey of Child and Adolescent Well-Being
NSPCC	National Society for the Prevention of Cruelty to Children
PCS	picture communication symbols
RAC	Research Advisory Committees

REB	Research Ethic Boards
REC	Research Ethic Committees
RNIB	Royal National Institute of the Blind
SACG	*South Asia Coordinating Group on Action against Violence against Children*
SAIEVAC	South Asian Initiative to End Violence against Children
SDGs	Sustainable Development Goals
UCR	Uniform Crime Reports
UNCRC	United Nations Convention on the Rights of the Child
UNICEF	United Nations Children's Fund
UPIAS	Union of the Physically Impaired against Segregation
WHO	World Health Organization

AUTHOR BIOGRAPHIES

Dr **Deborah Fry** is a Lecturer in Child Protection and co-leads the Safe Inclusive Schools Network at the University of Edinburgh, Moray House School of Education.

Dr **Patricia Lannen** is the UBS Optimus Foundation's program director for child protection and has been involved in research on vulnerable children for fifteen years.

Dr **Jennifer Vanderminden** is an Assistant Professor of Sociology at the University of North Carolina, Wilmington.

Dr **Audrey Cameron** worked as a Research Fellow in Child Protection (Disabilities) at the University of Edinburgh (2013–15) and is a very active member of the Deaf community.

Tabitha Casey is Project Manager for the Safe Inclusive Schools Network at the University of Edinburgh, Moray House School of Education.

FOREWORD

Claudia Cappa, UNICEF

Millions of children around the world experience the worst kinds of rights violations. Millions more children, not yet victims, are inadequately protected against them. Children with disabilities are particularly vulnerable to abuse and exploitation. They are among the most likely to be subjected to bullying and sexual violence, to experience neglect and to be deprived of family care. They are also among the least likely to get an education, to access services and to be reached by violence-prevention initiatives.

Sadly, these rights violations are under-recognised. This is mainly due to a shortage of sound data on the lives of children with disabilities and those who care for them. Such shortage has many causes. In some cases, it has stemmed from lack of capacity and resources for data collection and, in other cases, from insufficient investments in improving measurement. Research and data collection on children with disabilities has long been affected by the adoption of very narrow (and often stigmatising) definitions of disability. Furthermore, collecting data on sensitive child protection issues presents serious methodological and ethical challenges, and different research approaches have been developed, including the use of diverse measurement tools and data-collection protocols.

This combination of factors has often led to the collection of data of varying scope and quality, especially in low- and middle-income countries. It has also raised important questions about the risks and ethical issues that arise when the data-collection process involves vulnerable children. Ultimately, the lack of rigorous evidence and robust data has long compromised the ability of governments and the international community to accurately document the widespread nature of child protection violations against children with disabilities, to support planning and budgeting for services and to inform the development of effective policies.

In the 2030 Agenda for Sustainable Development, the world's governments call for reliable data that goes beyond averages to ensure that no one is left behind. Solid data on which to act and with which to measure progress, including on crucial issues – such as violence against children – was missing from previous international commitments. For this to happen, existing knowledge gaps must be documented and promising research methods and tools have to be promoted.

It is to that end that this book is dedicated. It provides a comprehensive overview of examples from around the world of research that has been conducted to unveil the extent and nature of violence against children with disabilities. It covers what we know, and where the gaps are. Most importantly, it gives guidance on how to conduct ethical and sound research in this area.

I am confident this book will encourage new research and stimulate much needed action to document child protection violations worldwide. We now have another powerful resource on which we can rely to strengthen the knowledge that makes progress possible and societies safe for all children.

INTRODUCTION

In 2006, the UN Secretary General published a landmark report that highlighted the state of violence against children globally and put violence against children on the agenda (Pinheiro, 2006). A decade later, some progress has been made to understand how to stop violence against children before it ever starts and how to improve our responses. Yet, much more work is still required. Violence against children is still highly prevalent. Recent research has discovered that more than one billion children, or half of all the children in the world, are exposed to violence every year (Hillis *et al.*, 2016). Research also shows that children with disabilities are at an increased risk to violence from parents and caregivers, other adults as well as peers compared to children without disabilities (Jones *et al.*, 2012).

Violence is multifaceted and includes physical, sexual and emotional violence and neglect by caregivers and other adults, witnessing violence between adults as well as experiencing violence by peers and children (Krug *et al.*, 2002). These forms of violence occur in homes, schools, institutions and in the community (Pinheiro, 2006). What these forms of violence share is their potential for lifelong health, well-being and social consequences for children and adults. The consequences for children experiencing abuse and neglect are far-reaching and include impacts on mental and physical health and well-being, social withdrawal, increased risk behaviours, aggression and exposure to further violence as well as impacts on education and employment (Fry, 2012; Gilbert *et al.*, 2009; Margolin and Gordis, 2004). Childhood experiences of violence also have an economic cost and undermine the social and economic development of communities and nations (Fry *et al.*, 2016; Hillis *et al.*, 2015).

Violence is defined from Article 19 of the United Nations Convention on the Rights of the Child (UNCRC) as 'all forms of physical or mental violence, injury or abuse, neglect or negligent treatment, maltreatment or exploitation, including sexual abuse' (United Nations General Assembly, 1989). Furthermore, Article 16 of the United Nations Convention on the Rights of Persons with Disabilities (CRPD) mandates policymakers to 'take all appropriate legislative, administrative, social, educational and other measures to protect persons with disabilities, both within and outside the home, from all forms of exploitation, violence and abuse' (United Nations General Assembly, 2006). Recently published global estimates show that a minimum of 50% of children in Asia, Africa and North America were victims of some form of violence in the past year, and that globally approximately one billion children ages 2–17 years have experienced such violence (Hillis *et al.*, 2016). Evidence focusing primarily on the US also highlights that children with disabilities are more likely to be abused than children without disabilities (Jones *et al.*, 2012).

With these shocking numbers, policymakers and practitioners are asking what causes violence against children with disabilities and how do we stop it? Both policymakers and practitioners want to know the *scope and magnitude* of violence against children with disabilities and also what strategies for prevention and response are *evidence-based*. Both of these areas require research, and while there is growing research to date on violence against children with disabilities no publication – until now – has sought to synthesise this evidence base for lessons learned on how to best address the ethical and methodological challenges of conducting research in this area.

The Sustainable Development Goals: An inclusive global agenda

The Sustainable Development Goals (SDGs), often called the 2030 Agenda, are a universal set of seventeen goals, 169 targets with 231 global indicators that UN member states adopted in 2015 and will be expected to use to frame their agendas and political policies over the next fifteen years (United Nations General Assembly, 2015). The SDGs expand a previous set of goals and targets called the Millennium Development Goals (MDGs), which were agreed by governments in 2001 and expired in 2015. The drafting of the SDGs was one of the most participatory global agenda-setting exercises to date with an open working group consisting of seventy countries in addition to eleven thematic and eighty-three national consultations and a global survey with more than seven million responses (United Nations General Assembly, 2014). The SDGs are important because not only will they frame upcoming policy and programming initiatives at national, regional and global levels, but also they represent areas where further funding from governments, research funding bodies, global agencies and the private sector will be focused.

Neither people with disabilities nor violence against children were referenced in the previous MDGs. This means they were excluded from many important development initiatives and funding streams around the world. By contrast, persons with disabilities are referenced directly eleven times in the SDGs. The inclusive phrasing of many goals and targets also makes them applicable for people with disabilities, such as those referencing 'for all' or 'all women and men' or 'all children' (IDDC, 2016). Even without any such references, all goals and targets will be applicable to children with disabilities because of the 2030 Agenda's overarching principle of leave no one behind. All SDGs are also linked to the United Nations CRPD Articles, and this should serve as a guiding framework for policy and programming (IDDC, 2016).

For the first time, several violence-prevention indicators are included in the SDGs. This is with the recognition that none of the goals for children can be met if children are not safe. The SDGs include protecting children from violence as a distinct and cross-cutting priority across all goals. Specifically, five goals and eleven targets address violence and abuse, trafficking, sexual and other types of exploitation, harmful practices such as child marriage and the worst forms of child labour including children in armed forces (SACG and SAIEVAC, 2016). In addition, the goals focus on the promotion of safe public spaces including safe, non-violent and inclusive learning environments.

According to General Assembly Resolution 68/261, which details the SDG targets and indicators, data should be disaggregated in line with the SDG commitment, where relevant, by income, sex, age, race, ethnicity, migratory status, *disability* and geographic location, or other characteristics, in accordance with the Fundamental Principles of Official Statistics (United Nations General Assembly, 2014). Furthermore, the use of a new monitoring framework and set of indicators, as identified through the SDGs, will require additional capacity strengthening and support for many countries in order to improve the evidence-based approach, including data disaggregation, to tracking progress on the SDGs related to violence against children.

Definitions

There is no accepted universal definition of disability (Palmer and Harley, 2012). The World Health Organization (WHO) defines disability as:

> ... the interaction between individuals with a health condition (e.g. cerebral palsy, Down syndrome and depression) and personal and environmental factors (e.g. negative attitudes, inaccessible transportation and public buildings, and limited social supports) (WHO and World Bank, 2011).

Known as the bio-psycho-social model, this explicitly defines disability as the interaction between impairment and the social and physical environment. It is a hybrid definition between the medical model of disability, which focuses solely on individual impairments, and the social model of disability, which argues that exclusion occurs not because of the individual's inability to fit in with their surrounding environment but because of society's inability to include them (Palmer and Harley, 2012). In the 1970s, the Union of the Physically Impaired against Segregation (UPIAS) manifesto made a distinction between impairment – the lost or limited functioning experienced by an individual – and the exclusion and barriers that people face because of the way societies are organised (UPIAS, 1975). Defining disability in this way is the key to identifying the barriers within society and communities for people with disabilities and addressing them. The benefits of the social model of disability allow for a more holistic model than the medical model to discuss/view disability. In addition, this model also highlights how disability varies by social and physical environment and importantly allows for a more nuanced analysis of its relation to victimisation.

There are many debates about the use of language and differing terminologies. We use the term 'children with disabilities' as it recognises the *person first*. This is also the term adopted by the United Nations in its *State of the World's Children* (UNICEF, 2013), the CRPD, and is the term adopted in the SDGs, a global agenda for inclusion and prevention of violence against children, among other global issues, that will direct international and national policy and practitioner initiatives in these areas for *all countries* over the next fifteen years.

However, this terminology has been criticised for assuming 'that the *person* has the disability', whereas 'disabled person' is said to acknowledge that a person is *disabled* by societal barriers (Chapman, 2013). This terminology is standard in the UK, where 'disabled children and young people' or 'deaf and disabled children and young people' are primarily used (Stalker *et al.*, 2015; Stalker *et al.*, 2010). The authors fully respect the importance of language when talking about disability and use the term 'children with disabilities' in this book in recognition of the diversity of the population. Further, as terms such as 'moderate' or 'severe' to describe 'degrees' of disability are rooted in a medical model perspective, these are mentioned in this book only when the source material has made these distinctions. We will also use the distinction between deaf – referring to a hearing loss – and Deaf, which refers to identity with a distinct cultural community whose first or preferred language is sign language (Woodward, 1972). Finally, the term 'children' refers to those under the age of eighteen as defined by the UN Convention on the Rights of the Child (United Nations General Assembly, 1989). Violence against children refers to acts of physical, sexual and emotional abuse, neglect and exploitation as defined by the UNCRC (ibid.). The terms violence and abuse will be used interchangeably.

Overview of the book

This book explores the ethical, methodological, and practical challenges in conducting child protection research with children with disabilities across three main themes: what we know and the limits to our current knowledge; the practical concerns and challenges faced by researchers in the field; and some strategies and approaches to overcome these challenges in order to protect children. This edited volume draws upon examples of international research in both child protection and disability fields and explores how best to include children with disabilities as participants in research, while keeping their protection as the overarching and primary goal.

Chapter 1 explores our current evidence base on the prevalence, consequences and research related to child protection and disability. Data from around the world highlights how children with disabilities are at greater risk of experiencing violence when compared to children without disabilities with the majority of the studies coming from high-income countries. Studies that do exist show barriers in accessing response and preventative services. The Sustainable Development Goals (SDGs) have made a commitment to inclusion of children with disabilities in all strategies to prevention violence. However, governments and practitioners require data to measure progress against key recommendations and obligations to fulfil these goals. This chapter sets the stage for the remaining chapters of this book, which highlight the ethical and methodological challenges with planning, collecting, analysing and disseminating research in order to improve data-collection efforts for preventing and responding to violence against children with disabilities.

Chapter 2 delves into an overview of data sources on violence against children with disabilities, primarily from the US, as well as the specific methodological and ethical challenges associated with research on child protection and disability. The use of data in making violence against children with disabilities more visible is vital to better protect children. A majority of research indicates that children with disabilities face disproportionately high rates of violence, but there is a great deal of variability in the data type, quality and design, leading to inconsistent results. The extent and exact nature of this relationship remains poorly understood because of methodological and ethical challenges associated with collecting this type of data on this vulnerable and often marginalised population. Data sources on child victimisation and disability include child protection service reports, agency data and self-reports. The challenges associated with collecting, analysing and inferring from each type of victimisation data are exacerbated when focusing on children with disabilities specifically. Some of these issues include contact with potential reporters, disclosure rates, unrecognised signs and symptoms of abuse, if the child is believed, and whether or not the report is substantiated.

Chapter 3 focuses on the topic of informed consent and provides examples, many from the UK, of how to make this inclusive for children with disabilities. Informed consent is a vital part of the research process, and as such entails more than merely obtaining a signature on a form. The challenge for researchers is to engage with potential participants and enable them to achieve a level of confidence in making an informed decision about whether or not to contribute to a study. There is an urgent need to include the views children with disabilities in child protection research and to develop a better understanding of what informed consent means to them. For some, this means providing information about the research study in ways that are more accessible. Therefore, in this chapter, a number of practical suggestions are offered that researchers might want to consider when they are looking to work with children with disabilities in their research activities. The benefits of using a dialogic approach (Pollard *et al.*, 2009) to informed consent are also explored.

Chapter 4 highlights case studies of actual research from around the world. Based upon interviews with researchers who have conducted research on violence against children with disabilities, these case studies provide never before presented reflections on the challenges and lessons learned from conducting research in this area. Drawing on published works as well as interviews with researchers, we build a timely summary of good practices, while also highlighting methodological and research gaps in need of further attention. The chapter includes studies, some recently completed, some still ongoing from the US, the UK, Switzerland, Hong Kong, Burundi and Uganda. Studies were chosen with a variety of different methodologies, including longitudinal studies, evaluations of prevention programmes, as well as those that focused on experiences of victims with the support they received. Some of the findings explored in this chapter are: the need to include specific research expertise on disability as well as on violence to tackle a highly complex and ethically challenging issue; the importance of close collaboration with implementers to create trust, and have a solid referral system in place that is competent to deal with victims with disabilities; and the need to understand better how to assess the potential ethical risks of research.

Chapter 5 provides concrete guidance for conducting research on child protection and disability based on all the data gathered for this book. This chapter explores ethical issues arising and includes the need to balance respondents' right to participation while maintaining the highest level of child protection and ensuring the benefits to respondents or communities of documenting violence against children with disabilities are greater than the risks. Comprehensive training covering the basics of child protection and disability, the study protocol, safeguarding and referral pathways, safety for researchers as well as quality assurance of the data should be provided for all members of the research team including interpreters. Finally, research should also be conducted in such a way so as to maximise benefit to survivors of violence, participants and the community. Chapter 6 concludes the book by summarising the findings from the preceding chapters, and makes recommendations to ensure children with disabilities are included and protected in future violence research.

CHAPTER 1

Violence against children with disabilities: Evidence from around the world

Deborah Fry
Lecturer in Child Protection, Moray House School of Education, University of Edinburgh

Introduction

Data from around the world highlights how children with disabilities are at increased risk of experiencing all forms of violence when compared to their peers without disabilities. According to the UNCRC definition 'violence against children' (United Nations General Assembly, 1989) includes violence perpetrated by adults or other children and young people in a variety of settings including the home, schools, institutions and in the community (Pinheiro, 2006).

Despite the increased vulnerability of children with disabilities to experiencing violence, very little research has been conducted on child protection and disability and most of this research comes from high-income countries. Studies that do exist show barriers in accessing care and preventative responses. Recent global and regional recommendations were made for children with disabilities to be made visible in all strategies to tackle violence against children, emphasising both the need for them to be included in general violence-prevention initiatives and in disability-specific ones. The SDGs present an opportunity to take forward many of these recommendations over the next fifteen years as part of national and global policy agendas. However, these global, regional and national commitments require data to measure progress against key recommendations and obligations. This chapter sets the stage for the remaining chapters of this book that highlight the ethical and methodological challenges with planning, collecting,

1

analysing and dissemination in order to improve data-collection efforts for preventing and responding to violence against children with disabilities.

Prevalence of violence against children with disabilities

Globally, 150 million children are estimated to be living with a disability, the majority of whom are in low- and middle-income countries (LMICs) (WHO and World Bank, 2011). Data on the prevalence of violence against children with disabilities is limited, especially in LMICs. A recent meta-analysis of seventeen studies of violence against children with disabilities from high-income countries has shown that children with disabilities are three to four times more likely to be abused than their peers without disabilities (Jones *et al.*, 2012). The meta-analysis concluded that 26.7% of children with disabilities are victims of more than one type of violence in their lifetime. More than 20% experience physical violence and nearly 14% experience sexual violence (Jones *et al.*, 2012). This echoes results from an earlier US study of all the child protection case records in Nebraska, which found that children with disabilities were 3.4 times more likely to be abused than their peers without disabilities, with incidence rates of 31% and 9% respectively (Sullivan and Knutson, 2000). In Asia, a large study of 5,841 school-aged children in Hong Kong also reported a higher prevalence of child maltreatment among children with disabilities compared to their peers without disabilities (Chan *et al.*, 2014).

These findings are replicated in LMICs: in South Africa, for example, it has been discovered that children with physical disabilities are three to four times more likely to be abused than children without disabilities (Lamprecht, 2003). The Good School Study in Uganda, an evaluation of a school-based violence-prevention programme, randomly sampled approximately 3,800 children and adolescents aged 11–14 from forty-two primary schools in Luwero District. Among those in the control arm (n = 1,737), 84% of children with disabilities had experienced some form of violence at school in the past week compared to 54% of children without disabilities (Kuper *et al.*, 2016). This study also found that girls with disabilities experienced twice as much sexual violence versus girls without disabilities (Devries *et al.*, 2014). For boys, levels of sexual violence were nearly double those of boys without disabilities, but given the low prevalence of sexual violence in boys overall this difference was not statistically significant in the findings. Levels of emotional violence and neglect were noted to be similar between boys and girls with and without disabilities (Devries *et al.*, 2014; see Chapter 4 for more on this study).

There are several methodological issues involved in measuring the prevalence of violence against children, and research has shown that some of the variance between study findings may in fact be due to methodological issues (Pereda *et al.*, 2009). Some of the key difficulties in measurement can be found in the definitions of both disability and violence and in questions asked, the sampling designs, the age of the respondent and the type of study conducted. Also, for the first time, this book presents emerging findings that show the importance of who is asked about disability and time variance in measuring the prevalence of disability in a longitudinal study using parent–child dyads (see Chapter 4).

Evidence from a global meta-synthesis of 111 studies on physical abuse found that studies using a broad definition of child physical abuse, those that measured physical abuse across childhood (from 0–18 years) and research that included several questions on physical abuse led to higher self-reported prevalence rates (Stoltenborgh *et al.*, 2013). The number of questions asked and measuring across childhood also increased reporting of sexual abuse according to another global meta-analysis of 217 studies on child sexual abuse (Stoltenborgh *et al.*, 2011). However, for measuring emotional abuse prevalence, a global meta-analysis of studies found that type of instrument (face to face vs paper-and-pencil questionnaires among other approaches), whether or not the study used validated instruments, the number of questions or the sample size did not significantly impact on prevalence estimates (Stoltenborgh *et al.*, 2012). One of the only methodological considerations that led to underreporting for emotional abuse was sampling design with lower reported prevalence rates in randomised studies than those using convenience samples (Stoltenborgh *et al.*, 2012). In Chapter 2, we explore some of these key methodological challenges and the specific aspects that impact on the measurement of the prevalence of violence against children with disabilities.

Studies show that children with disabilities are vulnerable to many different forms of violence. There are many reasons for this increased vulnerability including: close and often intimate proximity to adults who act as caretakers; some physical and communication impairments that make it more difficult for children to disclose experiences of violence; legal and criminal justice systems, because of burden-of-proof standards, which make it more difficult to prosecute perpetration of violence against children with disabilities; and stigma and social norms that create environments where children with disabilities are discriminated against and are more isolated from potential protective factors.

In a qualitative study from Ethiopia, children with disabilities told their stories of experiencing neglect, forced labour and abandonment (Boersma, 2008). Research by Save the Children and Handicap International in Burundi, Madagascar, Mozambique and Zanzibar highlighted the increased vulnerability of children with disabilities to sexual violence (Save the Children and Handicap International, 2011). In a national survey of deaf adults in Norway, girls were twice as likely to be victims of sexual abuse, and boys three times as likely, as peers who had no disability (Kvam, 2000).

Recent research undertaken by Terre des Hommes in three countries in East Africa also highlights the increased violence against children with disabilities (Stöpler, 2007). In Kenya 15–20% of children with disabilities were exposed to severe levels of physical and sexual violence, with girls with learning disabilities being particularly vulnerable (ibid.) This is comparable to two studies from the Philippines showing an increased risk for sexual violence of children with disabilities (Terol, 2009; Hulipas, 2005).

Research has also shown that children with particular forms of impairment may be more at risk than others. Those with communication impairments, behavioural disorders, learning disabilities and sensory impairments are most vulnerable to maltreatment (Stalker and McArthur, 2012). In Uganda, children who self-reported having difficulties with self-care or communication were significantly more likely to mention severe injuries and sexual violence perpetrated by school staff compared to children without these difficulties (Kuper et al., 2016). These studies also highlight how disclosure is often delayed with most violence experiences of children who lack communication skills (mostly those with 'moderate' intellectual difficulties) being discovered only through noticeable symptoms such as a dishevelled appearance, physical marks, crumpled hair, soiled clothing and an unusually distressed condition (Terol, 2009).

International research has shown that non-verbal disclosure is not unique to children with disabilities. A recent qualitative study conducted in the UK on disclosure found that the majority of young adults who experienced violence during childhood attempted to disclose through their actions that they were experiencing violence during childhood but that adults often did not 'hear' or act upon these disclosures (Allnock and Miller, 2013; Taylor *et al.*, 2015a). Research has highlighted that children with disabilities may not disclose violence as frequently as their peers because of a number of barriers (Stalker and McArthur, 2012) (see Chapter 2 for a discussion of these factors). In these cases, the risk factors for violence, especially sexual violence, are compounded including the vulnerability of the child combined with increased accessibility to time alone with the child (most of these children were not in school) and delayed or non-disclosure because of the child's disability.

Responding to violence against children: The need for inclusive child protection systems

Despite the increased vulnerability of children and young people with disabilities to child maltreatment, very little research has been conducted on child protection and disability and most of this research comes from high-income countries. In a survey of seventy-three Area Child Protection Committees in the UK, Cooke and Standen (2002) found that, following case conferences (where child protection concerns are interrogated by the multidisciplinary team and which should include representation from family), children with disabilities were 'significantly' less likely than children without disabilities to be placed on child protection registers or have protection plans put in place. There is evidence internationally that the abuse of children with disabilities often goes undetected and, even when suspected, may be underreported (Kvam, 2004; Hershkowitz *et al.*, 2007).

In many countries, children with disabilities continue to be placed in institutions, as highlighted by the global UN Study on Violence against Children (Pinheiro, 2006). The care provided in institutions is often insufficient because standards of appropriate care for children with disabilities are lacking or are not monitored and enforced (UNICEF, 2013). Qualitative research in Northern Ireland involved interviews with sixty-three children and young people with disabilities in out-of-home care, their parents and support professionals, and found that the process of admission into foster care or residential care was often traumatic for the child, and that many were placed in care due to abuse or neglect, but few had access to therapeutic and counselling services in care (Kelly *et al.*, 2016). Under the Convention on the Rights of the Child (UNCRC), children with and without disabilities have the right to be cared for by their parents (Article 7) and not to be separated from their parents unless this is deemed by a competent authority to be in the child's best interest (Article 9). The CRPD reinforces this in Article 23, which states that where the immediate family is unable to care for a child with disabilities, State parties must take every measure to provide alternative care within the extended family or community (UNICEF, 2013). As a result, there is a global movement by family and relatives to promote deinstitutionalisation and care of children.

Child protection response often involves complex decision-making environments characterised by incomplete information. Research has shown that when working on issues related to child protection and disability, professionals may struggle in key areas (Kelly and Dowling, 2015). Working with children with communication impairments is seen as particularly challenging (Stalker *et al*, 2010; Taylor *et al*, 2014). The diagnostic system for assessing significant risk may also be broader and less accurate for children with disabilities than for children without disabilities (Taylor *et al.*, 2014). Professionals highlight that the difficulty in assessing risk is due in part to children with disabilities being more dependent on support from parents/carers and their greater vulnerability as a result, increased parental stress and complex family environments, and having multiple carers and care in different settings (ibid.).

In relation to thresholds, or when something moves from being an initial child protection concern to action within the child protection system, there is increasing evidence that professionals may apply higher thresholds for triggering a child protection response than are used with children without disabilities (Taylor *et al.*, 2014; Stalker *et al.*, 2010; Kelly and Dowling, 2015). In part this had been explained by a tendency of professionals to over-empathise with the parent and to be more tolerant of some behaviours than they would be of parents of children without disabilities (Stalker *et al.*, 2010). Research highlights that while interagency working is very positive in providing support around complex cases there is often very little opportunity for professionals to reflect on practice (Munro, 2011) particularly in relation to child protection and disability (Taylor *et al.*, 2014).

Preventing violence against children with disabilities

The landmark UN study on violence against children highlighted that 'no violence against children is justifiable. All violence against children is preventable' (Pinheiro, 2006). Furthermore, this report led to a thematic study on the issue of violence against children with disabilities, which concluded that while all children are at risk those with disabilities are at significantly increased risk (UNICEF, 2005). Recommendations were made for children with disabilities to be made visible in all strategies to tackle violence against children, emphasising both the need for them to be included in general violence-prevention initiatives and in disability-specific ones (Pinheiro, 2006).

In the UN general comment on children with disabilities from the Committee on the Rights of the Child, the obligations of governments include providing appropriate care and responses in the home, schools and institutions: for example, by making provision for education and support for parents, adopting measures to reduce bullying and abuse in schools and ensuring appropriate training, staffing and standards of care in childcare institutions. In addition, governments should provide access to complaints mechanisms, effective sanctions against and removal of abusers, and systems for ensuring appropriate treatment and rehabilitation of children with disabilities who have experienced violence (United Nations Committee on the Rights of the Child, 2007).

The UN CRPD, ratified by 165 countries, also emphasises these protections and rights of children with disabilities through several articles. Articles 16 and 39 highlight the right to protection from violence and require that all prevention, protection, recovery and rehabilitation services, as well as investigative services, are age, disability and gender sensitive. Based on this, Article 23 introduces obligations for governments to provide information, support and services to families to prevent the neglect and abandonment of children with disabilities including protection from sexual exploitation and abuse (Article 34) and from torture or other cruel, inhuman or degrading treatment of children (Article 37). Finally, Article 12 requires that governments ensure children are empowered to express their views on these and other matters affecting them and to have their opinions taken seriously in accordance with age and maturity. Article 12 also strengthens access to justice, by ensuring that all stages of legal proceedings are sensitive and accessible to people, including children, with disabilities.

An eight-country regional consultation took place in 2014 called 'Stepping up Protection of Children with Disabilities in South Asia' hosted by the South Asian Initiative to End Violence Against Children (SAIEVAC). The consultation put forward twelve recommendations to inform the work of governments going forward in the region. Much of this work seeks to address the root causes of violence and to inform future work as part of the SDGs (see Introduction) and represents the first regional consultation specifically aimed at preventing violence against children with disabilities. These recommendations include:

1.   Laws and policies need to be inclusive and non-discriminatory. They should be disability friendly and implemented effectively. There should be sufficient budgetary allocations to implement these policies and laws. Disability education needs to be introduced in school curriculums.

2.   The services such as education, health and public services should be inclusive, disability friendly, of good quality and accessible for children with disabilities. All the service providers must respect the dignity of children with disabilities. Also, a reporting mechanism should be in place to reach the concerned authorities directly.

3.   Measures should be taken to raise awareness among people to change attitudes and ensure respectful communications using good-quality and accessible information. It may include resource centres, code of conduct and the use of media.

4.   Measures need to be taken to develop skills and competencies of parents and professionals to work with children with disabilities.

5.   Opportunities need to be created for children with disabilities to participate at all levels including trainings on staying protected, economic empowerment and recreational activities.

6.   Children should also respect, support, treat equally and provide equal opportunities for children with disabilities.

7.   Families need to ensure equal participation of children with disabilities in social functions, family gatherings and other occasions. They should learn the issues and languages of the children with disabilities, provide a protective environment and pay more attention to the children with disabilities.

8.   Schools should have measures in place to protect children with disabilities from abuse and violence that involve the children's families.

Children with disabilities should be represented in decision-making in schools.

9. Private sectors should make their services accessible for all children with disabilities by removing language and infrastructure barriers. They should show sensitivity and have safety measures in place for children with disabilities.

10. Strict actions must be taken against those who commit violence against children with disabilities. Peace and security must be maintained in the region for the protection of the children with disabilities.

11. The technologies and equipment for supporting the children with disabilities should be improved and made available.

12. The governments, children and all other concerned actors should continue interaction and exchanges through regular consultations focusing on the rights and needs of children with disabilities at different levels (SAIEVAC, 2014).

Conclusion

In summary, children with disabilities are more vulnerable to abuse and neglect in both family and non-family settings and face greater challenges in either disclosing abuse or their abuse being discovered. This is due to aspects of their disability and to the lack of knowledge and skills of professionals in understanding what they may be trying to communicate through their disclosures or actions, as well as to the fact that this is a poorly researched area. There is also an increase in global commitments to ending violence against all children. However, these global, regional and national commitments require data to measure progress against key recommendations and obligations.

The following chapters highlight the ethical and methodological challenges with planning, collecting, analysing and dissemination in order to improve data-collection efforts for preventing and responding to violence against children with disabilities.

CHAPTER 2

Using data to make violence against children with disabilities visible: An overview of data sources, methodological challenges and ethical considerations

Jennifer Vanderminden

Assistant Professor of Sociology, University of North Carolina, Wilmington

Introduction

The use of data in making violence against children with disabilities more visible is vital to protect children and youth better. Data on violence in the lives of children with disabilities allows for a better understanding of the extent to which they experience violence, with the ultimate goal to inform policy and programmatic interventions. There is a wide range, in both type and quality, of data available on violence in the lives of children with disabilities. In this chapter, we will provide an overview of the data sources, largely from the US, and the methodological and ethical challenges we face in collecting this type of data.

As described in Chapter 1, a majority of research indicates that children with disabilities face disproportionately high rates of violence compared to their peers without disabilities (Jones *et al,.* 2012; Sullivan, 2009; Sullivan and Knutson, 2000; Spencer *et al.,* 2005; Harrell, 2012). The meta-analysis by Jones *et al.* (2012), which gathered data from sixteen research studies using random samples or whole population studies, found that prevalence rates of victimisation among children with disabilities varied widely, from 5% to 68%. While most data indicates higher rates, a number of studies indicate no difference in rates among children with and without disabilities (Benedict *et al.,* 1990; Leeb *et al.,* 2012), and yet others note that children with disabilities may be at lower risk for experiencing some forms of violence (Sedlak *et al.*, 2010). These discrepancies can be explained, in part, by the challenges associated with collecting data on children (Pereda *et al.*, 2009; Stoltenborgh *et al.*, 2011), specifically on children with disabilities on the topic of victimisation. An overview of the data sources follows, as well as the methodological and ethical challenges associated with researching violence in the lives of children with disabilities.

Overview of data sources

Epidemiological data sources on victimisation among children with disabilities include: official child protection services (CPS) reports, agency/administrative data, and survey data. To follow, we provide a brief description of these data sources along with examples of each. In addition to quantitative studies attempting to measure prevalence and incidence of victimisation we briefly discuss qualitative data sources on violence in the lives of children with disabilities.

Official CPS reports

CPS reports provide valuable information on victimisation in the lives of children with disabilities and should not be overlooked. The data from these reports contains details about those children who are known to social services and those who appear on the radar of agencies. In the US, CPS data is compiled in the National Child Abuse and Neglect Data System (NCANDS). The NCANDS database presents information on substantiated cases of child abuse and neglect in the US from all fifty states, based on CPS reports. One challenge associated with using this data – to determine risk among children with disabilities – is that, at last count, only thirty-one states reported the disability of the child (all adopting different definitions/criteria for disability) and there are no federal policies on reporting disability status in CPS reports. Therefore, information regarding the child's disability in CPS reports is highly variable across states. These issues are not unique to the United States.

Recent research in the UK found that only 31% of agencies/authorities have information on learning disabilities among children exposed to child sexual exploitation (Franklin *et al.*, 2015). Unfortunately, this research was limited to studying children with learning disabilities and did not explore other types of disabilities. In the UK, the NSPCC has complied child protection data from multiple sources available in the 'How safe are our children?' project (Bentley *et al.*, 2016). In the most recent report from the NSPCC, disability is mentioned as a risk factor, but no data is presented on differential risks for children with disabilities. In another study of children in West Sussex, Spencer *et al.* (2005) connect CPS reports to the health files of children, which is something that has not been done on a national scale in the United States to date.

In addition to the variability in reporting of disability in official reports, there are a number of other challenges and limitations surrounding the use of CPS data; this is something that will be examined in the Methodological challenges and Characteristics of disability sections.

Agency data

The National Incidence Study (NIS) is a congressionally mandated (US) national assessment of the incidence of maltreatment in the lives of children. The NIS suggests that using CPS data of known cases of child maltreatment only reveals the 'tip of the iceberg', given that the vast majority of cases go unreported. The NIS attempts to overcome this challenge by collecting information on child victimisation (mainly child maltreatment) from agencies including police, public health officials, juvenile probation officers, healthcare workers, teachers and social service agency workers (Sedlak *et al.*, 2010). Similar studies were conducted in Switzerland (Optimus Agency Study) and Canada (Canadian Incidence Study). The Canadian Incidence Study report notes that their measure of disability reflects the child welfare workers' knowledge of child functionality and limitations. This is problematic as it undercounts children with disabilities, as welfare workers do not consider child functionality as a routine part of their assessment/report (Public Health Agency of Canada, 2010).

The National Survey of Child and Adolescent Well-Being (NSCAW) is a nationally representative longitudinal study of children in the child welfare system in the US. Researchers have used this data to estimate the prevalence of disability within a sample of children already in the child welfare system (Helton and Bruhn, 2013). Other researchers have been creative with the use of agency data, combining information from the child welfare system with school data (Sullivan and Knutson, 2000), while others have linked child welfare data with databases such as the social service information system (Lightfoot *et al.*, 2011). Similar studies, highlighted earlier, have linked child protection registration reports and Child Health Special Conditions files in West Sussex, UK, to estimate the level of involvement in CPS among children with disabilities compared to children without disabilities (Spencer *et al.*, 2005).

The Uniform Crime Reports (UCR) is one of the primary sources of information on crime in the US. UCR is based on crimes reported to police and includes hate crimes against people with disabilities, but does not state the disability status of the victim for any crimes that do not have the 'hate crime' designation (e.g. assault, sexual assault, robbery).

One major limitation of using agency data to estimate violence in the lives of children is that it excludes those children who have not come to the attention of an agency/authority figure. Survey data indicates that only about one-third of maltreatment experienced in the past year is reported to an authority or agency (Finkelhor *et al.*, 2014a). The Optimus Study Switzerland found an even more alarming number – that only about 5% of cases were reported (Maier *et al.*, 2013). This limitation is likely exacerbated among children with disabilities, particularly those with high levels of dependency on caregivers, those with unique ways of communicating and among those who are socially isolated.

Survey research

Survey research has attempted to overcome the fact that much of the victimisation that children face goes unreported to authorities (Finkelhor *et al.*, 2014a); instead, it utilises self or parent (proxy) reports. Survey data allows researchers to obtain information on victimisation that may not have been disclosed to authorities, and would therefore be excluded from agency data and official reports. In addition, in some surveys we have the ability to ask about behaviours and experiences, even those that the child or parent did not conceptualise as violence or abusive. For examples, see the appendix in Finkelhor *et al.* (2014a).

Two major sources of survey research in the United States are the National Crime Victimization Survey (NCVS) and the National Survey of Children's Exposure to Violence (NatSCEV). The NCVS examines the experiences with crime among individuals in the US aged twelve and older (including individuals with disabilities). Unfortunately, the NCVS does not ask about experiences with child abuse, sexual abuse or kidnapping.

In addition, since the NCVS is a survey about crime, those experiences with violence that may not be considered as criminal behaviour may go underreported.

In the three waves of NatSCEV studies, researchers asked caregivers of children aged 0–9 years and youth aged 10–17 to report on the child's experiences with maltreatment in childhood (Finkelhor *et al.*, 2014a). NatSCEV includes caregiver reports about their child's experience with victimisation for children under the age of ten, in order to include the experiences of these children even before the children are able to participate themselves (ibid.). A limitation of this is that parents may not know about their child's experience with victimisation – this may be especially true for children with disabilities. Using the Juvenile Victimization Questionnaire (JVQ), the researchers were able to obtain information on fifty-four forms of victimisation. Disability status is reported in NatSCEV by the caregivers' reports of their child's conditions. Nearly 17% of the children in the NatSCEV (I) survey had a disability (Turner *et al.*, 2011).

Similar research in the UK also used the JVQ to examine the extent to which children are exposed to victimisation within the home, school and community (Radford *et al.*, 2011). This study included parents and youths aged 11–17 years and added an additional young adult sample of those aged 18–24. Radford *et al.* measured parent and child disability including detail as to whether the disability limits activities.

Qualitative data sources

Qualitative data on violence in the lives of children with disabilities provides rich details often unavailable in quantitative (often survey) research. There are three main foci of qualitative inquiry in this field including the perspective of: the child's (often retrospectively), the caregiver(s) and the personnel who work with victims of abuse or children with disabilities.

The first type – on research with victims of abuse – is undertaken to understand the abuse experience better (Boersma, 2008; Hershkowitz *et al.*, 2007; Odell, 2011), the process of disclosing (Hershkowitz *et al.*, 2007), support received/needed (Franklin *et al.*, 2015) and the short- to long-term consequences of the abuse. In one stage of their investigation into violence in the lives of children with learning disabilities, Franklin *et al.* (2015) asked children and youth about why they had been referred to child protection and for their experiences with the services provided. In-depth interviews and focus groups also provide context to assist researchers in better understanding the environments and circumstances in which children are at highest risk.

Qualitative research on caregivers of children with disabilities is the second focus and provides information as to how the parent perceives risk, their experiences with the child welfare system, and outcomes for their children. In a US-based research study on children with autism, caregivers (n = 40) were interviewed about what factors they considered to place their children with autism at higher risk for victimisation and what factors they saw as being protective (Pfeffer, 2014). In research on caregivers of children who experienced sexual abuse, Bernard (1999) examined the intersectionality between race and disability in exposure to sexual abuse.

The third focus is on the process through with child welfare workers, health workers and education staff identify victimisation, work with/serve individuals with disabilities, make determination about abuse including substantiating abuse reports (Cooke and Standen, 2002), and the challenges they face in doing so (Mallen, 2011; Shannon and Tappan, 2011; Stalker *et al.*, 2015). In-depth interviews with child protection workers provide insights as to the experiences and challenges associated with protecting children with disabilities. Research in this area has established that child protection workers often have limited training and resources for dealing with children with disabilities (Kelly and Dowling, 2015; Oosterhoorn and Kendrick, 2001; Shannon and Tappan, 2011). Furthermore, research on CPS in a Midwestern state (in the US) found that very few agencies had formal policies for working with people with disabilities (Lightfoot and LaLiberte, 2006). This type of research also allows for the examination of biases and myths that exist among child welfare workers regarding children with disabilities and their families. Using vignettes, Manders and Stoneman (2009) found that child protection workers were more likely to empathise with parents of children with disabilities and attribute the abuse to characteristics of the child.

Using qualitative data to examine violence in the lives of children with disabilities can be challenging, even problematic for a few reasons. First, qualitative research often draws on small non-probability samples of children known to medical personnel/therapists, authorities or other service providers and often means that they are in contact with the researcher and therefore more likely to have access to services, someone to disclose to, etc. For studies specifically focusing on victimisation, only those who are known to researchers/authorities are eligible for inclusion in the study. This is problematic because researchers are unable to access those cases unknown to researchers/authorities and because it is likely that the experiences of those unknown to authorities are different in important ways. While this is also a problem in quantitative research designs, quantitative design using general population samples are able to access children who are not yet known to researchers/authorities.

Second, most qualitative research is conducted (necessarily) on small non-probability samples and therefore cannot be generalised beyond the sample (Brownlie *et al.*, 2007; Shannon and Tappan, 2011). (See the Challenges to drawing inferences section for additional information on challenges in making generalisations.)

Third, in research focusing on agency workers, care workers may be hesitant to disclose the full extent of the challenges, barriers, bias and processes that go into working with children with disabilities, since in-depth interviews and focus groups cannot guarantee anonymity.

Lastly, most in-depth interviews with victims are conducted retrospectively once the child has aged into adulthood (Kvam, 2004). Retrospective reports are problematic among all children and may be particularly so among children with specific types of disabilities. While this is clearly an issue in qualitative research on disability and victimisation, it is important to note that this is also a challenge in many quantitative research studies on this topic (e.g. Kvam, 2000).

Methodological challenges

There are methodological challenges related to identifying the incidence and prevalence of victimisation among all children. The following section will identify these challenges broadly and discuss the ways in which they are exacerbated when attempting to collect victimisation information on children with disabilities. These issues make it difficult to calculate accurate rates of victimisation, to test hypotheses (examine risk factors and outcomes) and to generalise to larger populations. These challenges are reflected in the great deal of variability in findings of the relationship between disability and victimisation (Jones *et al.*, 2012). This is likely a reflection of the difficulties in collecting data on violence in the lives of all children, methodological differences across studies and the ways in which disability and victimisation are conceptualised and operationalised. Studies employing agency data and using child welfare workers' accounts for measuring disability undercount both the extent of victimisation and disability for reasons that we will explore here.

The definitions of disability and victimisation used in previous research differ substantially depending on the research framework, the data available and the discipline within which they are defined (medicine, psychology, sociology, etc.). Victimisation and disability have also been measured in a variety of ways and using different samples, often yielding inconsistent results. Estimates of the prevalence of victimisation vary, as do those assessing the prevalence of disability. This type of data collection has important implications in terms of interpretation of the results and generalisability. Some sources of data look only at CPS reports (e.g. NCANDS; NSCAW; Spencer et al., 2005), which indicate they have been brought to the attention of a state agency.

All research is limited in terms of the ability to measure violence in the lives of children, as illustrated in the prior section on data sources. It is clear that when we measure victimisation through official reports we miss a great deal of the experiences of children. Official child protection agency data as well as self-reports raise questions about the accuracy and comprehensiveness of data/reports. This is particularly relevant for children with disabilities. In the US, just over thirty states gather information on child's disability as a part of the CPS report. The ways in which this information is collected varies across states (e.g. some states have a checkbox for child disability, others ask for detailed information about disability status, while others are aware of disability information only if it is mentioned in the case notes).

As mentioned in the Introduction, there is no universally accepted definition of disability. This lack of consensus is reflected in the considerable variation in defining and measuring disability across studies. Most research operationalises disability as a dichotomous yes/no for any disability or for specific disabilities (Jones et al., 2012). Some studies ask parents/caregivers about a diagnosis of a condition (Turner et al., 2011), others use definitions (often yes/no) put forward by the US Department of Education (Sedlak et al., 2010; Sullivan and Knutson, 2000), and yet more adopt measures of symptomology (Helton and Cross, 2011; Ouyang et al., 2008) or functionality (Dubowitz et al., 2011). One study in Uganda measured disability using the Washington Group 'Short set of questions', a tool that is based on the WHO framework provided in the Introduction and asks questions about the self-reported degree of difficulty that individuals have with doing activities such as self-care, communicating with others or walking (CDC, 2015; see Chapter 4). It is rare to measure disability by asking how a child interacts with their physical or social environment in victimisation research, however There is a lack of knowledge on and systematic assessment of standardised measures of disability, particularly within the field of child protection. Researchers in this field often rely on a medical model definition of disability and are unable to account for the personal and environmental factors and the interaction between the impairment and the personal and environmental factors (e.g. attitudes around mental illness, accessibility of education system). Research in this field would benefit from a consistent definition that allowed for comparison across studies and one that included more than a medical diagnosis/symptomology approach. Chapter 4 highlights some examples of how different researchers have resolved this.

Challenges to drawing inferences

We have identified two main challenges to drawing inferences about the relationship between disability and victimisation: time structure and sampling/population. In addition to the challenges outlined above, these two factors are limitations of much of the data on disability and victimisation; these are areas where we could certainly improve.

Time structure

One essential characteristic of all data sources is the time structure. This section looks at examples of data sources that are cross-sectional, panel and longitudinal designs. One of the reasons the time dimension is so crucial to the relationship of disability and victimisation is to determine which is the antecedent and which is the outcome. There are two sizeable bodies of literature on maltreatment and disability that imply causal processes in opposing directions. One line of research suggests that children with disabilities are at increased risk of maltreatment (Sullivan and Knutson, 2000; Sprang et al., 2005; Turner et al., 2009). Alternatively, other research shows that children who experience maltreatment are more likely to develop disabilities, including emotional and behavioural problems (Hildyard and Wolfe, 2002; Trickett and McBride-Chang, 1995; Appleyard *et al.*, 2005; Éthier *et al.*, 2004; Manly *et al.*, 2001). Another important consideration in terms of the time structure of the data is that disability might be noticeable/detected only later in life: for example, during primary school years. Importantly, some disabilities can be treated (e.g. physical impairment in early childhood that is treated with surgery and therapy) or may dissipate over time as the child grows/develops, so reporting of disability and victimisation may change over time for this reason as well.

Cross-sectional data

A majority of the available data on exposure to violence among children with disabilities is cross-sectional and therefore unable to address time order. Cross-sectional data is useful for understanding prevalence rates and correlation of victimisation at a single point in time, but is limited in terms of the conclusions we can draw on the relationship between disability and violence exposure.

Panel data

Panel data is useful for tracking trends over time and allowing for an assessment of changes in rates of victimisation. NatSCEV is a panel dataset with three nationally representative different samples of children ages 0–17 years old at three points in time. Likewise, the NIS datasets can be examined for changes over time in victimisation trends. Panel data, while beneficial for looking at variations in trends over time is unable to address the time order question. Some data sources, like NatSCEV, approximate time order by using recent victimisation experiences and by attempting to isolate the time of diagnosis of disability (to more than one year before).

Longitudinal data

Longitudinal data that includes measures of victimisation and disability is scarce. The Longitudinal Studies Consortium on Child Abuse and Neglect (LONGSCAN) and NSCAW are two primary sources of longitudinal data on this topic, but are both limited to high-risk children (for NSCAW all children are in the child welfare system). These longitudinal data sources allow for an evaluation of time order, but do not enable researchers to make generalisations beyond high-risk or child-welfare populations. This data allows researchers to examine changes over time within the individual on both disability and victimisation exposure/risk. Another limitation of these longitudinal designs is that the definitions of disability and diagnoses change over time (e.g. potential diagnoses of autism and Asperger's vary over time due to diagnostic criteria in the *Diagnostic and Statistical Manual of Mental Disorders* (DSM5)), making it difficult to compare conditions and variations in self-reports. An example of this is a case study presented in Chapter 4, which analysed correlations of disability measure (by multiple informants) over time and found very poor correlation between self-reports of disability.

A 2005 UNICEF report cites:

> Whether disabled due to violence within the family or within the community, once disabled the child who has already been a victim of violence, now becomes part of the population of disabled children all of whom are at increased risk of subsequent violence (Groce, 2005, p. 23).

It is likely that this is true and that the relationship between disability and violence is bidirectional, though we have not yet seen empirical research to test this hypothesis.

Sample and population

General population studies examining exposure to victimisation among children with disabilities that use random sampling designs and result in a sample representative of the population are particularly strong in terms of being able to estimate prevalence and in making inferences about the larger population. One of the limitations of general population studies is that they may be restricted in terms of ability to parse out specific types of disabilities that have a fairly low prevalence rate in the general population without a very large sample size (e.g. physical disabilities, conduct disorder). For example, using a single wave of the NatSCEV (I) data, researchers were unable to isolate the effects of conduct disorder as a risk factor for victimisation because of the relatively low prevalence rate of conduct disorder (Turner *et al.*, 2011). Most of the large-scale studies examining victimisation in the lives of children with disabilities are from a victimisation focus, and while they include disability information they are not designed to examine disability specifically. In data collected just to examine disability, oversampling children with disabilities allows researchers to examine the influence of disability while making inferences about the larger population. This type of data is scarce.

A number of the major sources of information on children rely on school samples (Good School Survey; Add Health; Global School-Based Health Surveys; Sullivan and Knutson, 2000, etc.). Children who are not in mainstream schools are less likely to be included in the general school population surveys, while children in schools catering specifically to those with disabilities may be more likely to be included in disability-specific research. It is important to note here that some research has identified boarding schools/institutions for children with disabilities as contexts in which children with disabilities are victimised at higher rates (Odell, 2011).

Many of the studies focusing on violence in the lives of children with disabilities are limited to samples of only children with disabilities (e.g. special schools or camps) (Reiter *et al.*, 2007). They allow an examination of the extent, frequency and type of violence in the lives of a subset of children with disabilities, but comparisons to children without disabilities cannot be made, nor a representative sample of children with disabilities. Other sources focus exclusively on children with abuse reports (e.g. NSCAW) and can include an examination of the type and prevalence of disabilities in a maltreated population, but comparisons to children without abuse reports is not possible. As mentioned earlier, qualitative data on the experiences of children with violence and the experiences of agency workers in working with children exposed to violence is crucial but often limited to non-probability samples. These respondents provide insights as to the experiences of those within the study but limits the generalisations beyond those groups that can be made. Nationally representative data repeated over time and with a design focus on both disability and victimisation is needed.

'Counted' in research: Who is included and who is left out?

Figure 2.1 illustrates the various pathways to which victimisation among children can become known to researchers. This figure traces the ways in which children with specific types of disabilities may be excluded, starting with contact with potential reporters, then moving into whether the victimisation was disclosed, if the disclosure was believed or if there were visible signs/symptoms of abuse, and lastly if the allegations were substantiated.

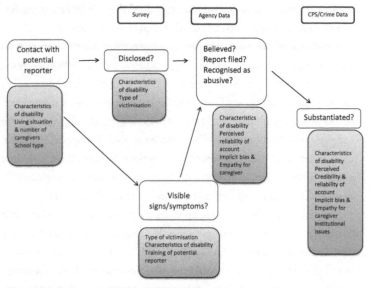

Figure 2.1: Pathways to inclusion in victimisation data.

Potential reporter

A promising first step in this process for all children is having contact with a potential reporter to possibly disclose to or to have the violence disclosed by someone else (e.g. potential reporter). For the purposes of being included in data on exposure to violence, this may be with a teacher, medical personnel, police officer, child protection worker or even a researcher. The likelihood of having contact with a researcher or an authority figure varies by type and characteristics of disability, and by living situation, including the number of caregivers. To follow, we review how each of these variables potentially impacts on contact with a reporter.

Research on violence in the lives of children often relies on children disclosing the abuse or neglect, and it is clear that many children never disclose their experiences to a researcher or authority. Some researchers argue that the elevated reports of victimisation among children with disabilities are still underestimates of the actual extent to which children with disabilities are victimised (Petersilia, 2001). While disclosure is a challenge for collecting victimisation data on all children, some argue that part of the reasons for these underestimations are the even lower rates of disclosure of victimisation among children with disabilities (Hershkowitz *et al.*,

2007; Petersilia, 2001). If the child has access to potential reporters, the next challenge is disclosure. Even among children with access to adults to whom they can do this, actually disclosing varies by a number of factors including the characteristics of the disability and the type of victimisation. Sometimes, even when confided in, adults do not 'hear' or understand the disclosure by children with disabilities, or do not believe the accusations against the parents/caregivers, etc. (Taylor *et al.*, 2015a; Allnock and Miller, 2013).

Visible signs and symptoms of abuse
Another way in which abuse can become known to authorities is through visible signs and symptoms of abuse, not necessarily requiring disclosure by the child (Wilczynski *et al.*, 2015). This could be through physical evidence such as bruises identified by doctors, to more behavioural signs or changes noticed by caregivers, therapists or teachers, etc. As with disclosure, these signs and symptoms frequently go undetected among all children. Knowing what signs and symptoms are associated with victimisation and which are genuinely accidents, reflecting other non-victimisation problems (mental health), or just typical child activities is a challenge. The signs of abuse being masked or going unrecognised are even more likely among children with disabilities. The accuracy with which signs and symptoms of abuse are reported likely varies by the type of victimisation, characteristics of disability and training of the potential reporter.

Among children who have contact with a potential reporter and then disclose or display visible signs/symptoms of victimisation, the next stage is the reaction by the potential reporter. Is the child believed? Are the signs recognised as abuse? Is the report filed? Unfortunately, both children with and without disabilities disclose abuse and are not believed or taken seriously. This is a societal problem and reflects an additional challenge to understanding the extent to which children are experiencing victimisation. This difficulty, while an issue for all research on violence in the lives of children, is especially problematic for children with disabilities. Research has demonstrated that while children with disabilities are disclosing (both verbally and other ways) they are not being believed or see no action taken on their behalf (Taylor *et al.*, 2015a). The reaction by an adult depends on a number of factors, including the characteristics of the disability, the perceived reliability of the account, implicit bias about disabilities and children with disabilities and empathy for the caregiver, as well as some systemic/institutional factors that can influence decision-making (e.g. do we have enough people to handle this case?).

There are several steps in order for abuse to be considered 'substantiated'. In many child protection systems data sources, the child has: had contact with a potential reporter; disclosed abuse or exhibited visible signs/symptoms that were recognised as abusive, and a report was filed. Yet we know from research that whether or not a report is substantiated is patterned by disability status (Manders and Stoneman, 2009) as well as characteristics of disability, perceived credibility/reliability of account, implicit bias/empathy for caregiver, and other institutional issues.

Characteristics of disability

At every point in Figure 2.1, the characteristics of the disability influence the likelihood of a child's victimisation experience becoming known, recognised and substantiated. In research aimed at investigating the type and prevalence of victimisation in the lives of children, those with disabilities – particularly children who are unable to communicate in typical ways – are often excluded (Cocks, 2008). Children with speech or hearing impairments and those with learning disabilities are less likely to be selected into the sample because of a lack of accessible options in general victimisation research (ibid.). Research that does not provide accessible options (interpreter, materials in braille, etc.) excludes children who are unable to communicate in typical ways (speaking, typing, etc.). Moreover, children with developmental delays and intellectual disabilities are often excluded for their inability to complete the research instrument on their own (Radford et al., 2011). This is clearly problematic as children who are unable to speak will likely also have fewer people to whom they are able to disclose experiences with violence. Disclosures to other potential reporters such as teachers and friends may be misunderstood or ignored (Taylor et al., 2015a).

Much of the epidemiological data on victimisation is focused on violence and not disability. This focus on victimisation results in narrow measures of disability, inaccessibility for many children with disabilities, and potentially small samples of children with specific types of disabilities. (See Sample and population section for more information.) These children are thought to be at increased risk of victimisation, making their exclusion from research particularly problematic.

In addition to reduced participation in research, children with communication impairments and those with more 'severe' disabilities, including intellectual disabilities and physical disabilities, are more likely to be socially isolated (Franklin *et al.*, 2015) and have limited interaction with others unless there is a clear mechanism in place for inclusion. In both social settings and in research, children with disabilities are more likely to be excluded if efforts are not made for inclusion (Cocks, 2008). This social isolation results in contact with fewer potential reporters to whom children could disclose victimisation experiences. Chapter 4 details a number of case studies that are making inclusion of children with disability in research a priority. Research on how cases become known to authorities has found that reports of victimisation for children are more likely to come from parents and teachers compared to social workers and healthcare professionals (Cooke and Standen, 2002). This may reflect exposure to potential reporters on whether or not the abuse is recognised, which we will detail later in this chapter. This may also reflect lower thresholds for a disclosure actually going into the system among parents and educators versus child protective worker and health professionals.

In a study of children seen in Norwegian emergency departments, Kvam (2000) examined the disability along with other risk factors in predicting sexual abuse. In this study, 'severe' disabilities are defined as 'children with severe hearing loss, severe visual handicap, mental retardation, severe orthopaedic disability, or multiple disabled (having more than one impairment)' (Kvam, 2000, p. 1,076). The results of this study indicate that children with 'severe' disabilities were underrepresented in the sexual abuse group, and this discrepancy can likely be explained through lower rates of disclosure. It is important to note that this research relies on a small sample of children with 'severe' disabilities. In another study using a sample drawn from the National Institute of Child Health and Human Development, researchers also found support for the notion that children with disabilities, especially more 'severe' disabilities, are less likely to disclose abuse. Among those who do disclose, the amount of time leading to disclosure is longer compared to children without disabilities (Hershkowitz *et al.*, 2007). Chapter 4 will describe how researchers conducting a study in Burundi made sure they included data on children with 'severe' disabilities.

Researchers have noted that, among children with some kinds of disabilities, victimisation may go unnoticed because of the child's condition (Kendall-Tackett *et al.*, 2005). In the study mentioned above, Kvam found that sexual abuse was frequently unrecognised among children with disabilities, especially children with 'severe' disabilities (Kvam, 2000). Further research has examined the extent of knowledge of physical symptoms of child sexual abuse, particularly among children with intellectual disabilities. Researchers found a lack of awareness and ability to identify symptoms of child sexual abuse, particularly among children with intellectual disabilities (Koetting *et al.*, 2012).

There are concerns surrounding the use of CPS reports like the NCANDS for measuring maltreatment, including how the reports are made, and the capabilities of the human agency associated with compiling these reports. Multiple studies have found that child welfare workers are less likely to pursue cases of maltreatment among children with disabilities, because characteristics of the disabilities were confused or considered to contribute to the abuse (Manders and Stoneman, 2009; Taylor *et al.*, 2014) and they lack confidence in working with children with disabilities (Taylor *et al.*, 2014). Manders and Stoneman (2009) conducted a study including eight vignettes to determine the impact of disability status on case outcomes in the CPS system. They found that CPS workers responded differently depending on the disability status of the child. Children with cerebral palsy were least likely to receive a substantiated report, as their injuries were interpreted as resulting from their disabilities rather than as indicators/outcomes of abuse (Manders and Stoneman, 2009). This study and another also found that social workers were more likely to empathise with parents of children with disabilities, particularly among those with behavioural problems (Manders and Stoneman, 2009; Brandon *et al.*, 2012). Therefore, it is possible that children with disabilities could be underrepresented in some high-risk maltreatment samples. Consistent with these findings, using in-depth interviews with child welfare workers, researchers found that abuse was often not recognised as abuse among children with disabilities and instead was attributed to the child's disability (Cooke and Standen, 2002; Nowak, 2015).

A study conducted in Austria, Germany and Switzerland (Niehaus *et al.*, 2013) on sexual abuse among adolescents and adults with intellectual disabilities examined the extent to which professionals (police, judges, prosecutors, forensic-psychiatric experts and social workers) would be subject to myths about disability and whether these myths could be detected in the case files. Similar to the concept of the 'rape myth', which was first introduced in the 1970s by sociologists (Schwendinger and Schwendinger, 1974) and feminists (Brownmiller, 1975) and has been extensively researched since then (Lonsway and Fitzgerald, 1994), myths about intellectual disability and sexual victimisation have also been described and documented (Senn, 1988; Dinos *et al.*, 2015). Such myths include, for example, assumptions that presumed unattractiveness will protect individuals with disabilities from sexual abuse or, on the other hand, that individuals with disabilities tend to behave in sexually suggestive or inappropriate ways in public, which may lead them to be more at risk of sexual abuse (Krüger *et al.*, 2014). In their study, Niehaus *et al.* (2013) investigated the effects of attitudes, knowledge and acceptance of myths in the assessment of case examples in relation to the credibility of the case. The effects of acceptance of myths on the actual criminal proceedings were tested using both quantitative and qualitative analysis of the case files. The results confirmed the presence of myths even in supposedly 'objective' case files documenting the court proceedings. The results further confirmed that even experienced professionals were subject to such myths (Niehaus *et al.*, 2013). Future efforts should increase our understanding of how these myths influence the research process, and the very outcome (Reiman, 2014).

Living situation and number of caregivers
Children who have few caregivers will also have fewer opportunities to have contact with a potential reporter, or a person with whom they have developed a trusting relationship to disclose to (Hibbard *et al.*, 2007). On the other hand, children with more caregivers may have more opportunities to disclose, but they may also be at increased risk of abuse (specifically emotional and sexual abuse) because of the increased number of people who have access to the child (Hibbard *et al.*, 2007; McCarthy and Thompson, 1996). This is particularly true among children with disabilities in need of assistance when dressing, bathing, etc. It may also be the case that children with disabilities have close contact with therapists, aides and other adults in ways that children without disabilities may not. The quality of relationships is likely more important than the

sheer number of caregivers. In a recent study of deaf children and children with disabilities, researchers found that having an interpreter with whom the child felt comfortable was crucial for disclosing abuse (Taylor et al., 2015a).

Children living in institutional settings such as group homes and specialised schools may have reduced access to potential reporters (both researchers and authorities) while at the same time institutional care could contribute to the vulnerability of children with disabilities (Helton and Cross, 2011; Westcott and Jones, 1999; Cambridge, 1999). This is particularly distressing as children in these circumstances face an increased risk of victimisation while at the same time have access to fewer potential people to report this victimisation to. According to the 'World report on violence against children':

> Violence against children in care and justice systems is legitimised by long-held attitudes and behaviours, and failures in both law and its implementation. At the time when the establishment of care institutions for children in disadvantaged and marginal groups was a preferred social policy, corporal punishment was almost universally endorsed for the discipline and control of unruly children. This effectively meant that institutionalised children were exposed to a brutal regime and to frequent violence (Pinheiro, 2006, pp. 180–1).

Type of victimisation

The type of victimisation influences the very likelihood that it will be disclosed, as well as the visibility of the symptoms. According to self and parent reports, emotional abuse, neglect and physical abuse are least likely to be known to authorities (Finkelhor et al., 2014a). It is unclear how disclosures by victimisation type also vary by disability. The social context in which the victimisation takes place likely plays an important role in the ways in which individuals define specific types of victimisation and appropriate reactions to violence against children with disabilities. It is likely that these disclosures are patterned and may be influenced by the level of understanding of the child (recognised as wrong), the level of dependency on the perpetrator, social context and access to a safe person to disclose to.

In returning to the question of how children are included in research as victims of violence/abuse, if victimisation is disclosed to researchers (such as in a telephone survey) the child is then 'counted' in the study as belonging to the victimised group of children. For authorities/official report data, the process then depends on whether the child is believed – if there is evidence to support the claim, and the claim is substantiated. The top of Figure 2.1 shows the point at which children are included in each type of data on victimisation (survey, agency, CPS).

Many types of victimisation do not have outward signs/symptoms such as broken bones or bruises but instead are associated with mental health and behavioural changes (Wilczynski et al., 2015). These types of abuses are difficult to identify in the general population of children, and are particularly challenging to spot among children with disabilities. Some combinations of abuse and disability type may be especially challenging to identify signs of abuse: for example, a child who has both a physical disability and does not communicate verbally. Physical signs of abuse may be masked by characteristics of the physical disability and behavioural/verbal signs/symptoms may also go unnoticed because of the child's communication style. Some symptoms of emotional abuse may be more difficult to identify among children who have a hard time engaging in social settings: for example, children on the autism spectrum.

Training of potential reporters

The extent to which a reporter is trained in identifying symptoms of abuse is incredibly important, particularly among children with disabilities. Relationships in which abusive situations are most likely to be recognised are close and trusting, and in which the adult has understanding of the specific type of disability (Taylor et al., 2015a), signs of abuse and perhaps most importantly an understanding of the specific child. Unfortunately, many adults working with children are not trained on the warning signs of abuse, on disabilities or how to work with children with disabilities (Franklin et al., 2015; Orelove et al., 2000). One US study, for example, found that only 6% of caseworkers and law enforcement personnel surveyed felt they were 'very knowledgeable' about 'how to respond to an abused child with disabilities' (Orelove et al., 2000). As described in Chapter 4, case studies in the

UK, Uganda and Burundi highlighted the particular importance of training reporters when doing research in a global context.

Reliability of account

Allegations of abuse of children with disabilities are less likely to be reported to authorities or pursued by authorities: once reported the accused are less likely to be prosecuted because 'officials hesitate to rely on the testimony of a person with a developmental disability' (Petersilia, 2001, p. 655). Among children with intellectual disabilities, authorities may also be unsure if the experiences of the child were abusive, or simply typical care-giving behaviour (e.g. bathing, toileting). The lack of sexual education among children with intellectual disabilities contributes to this issue (Cooke and Standen, 2002; Franklin *et al.*, 2015). Not having the appropriate knowledge of what is acceptable touch and what is abuse, as well as the vocabulary to talk about these behaviours/experiences, also inhibits disclosure (Franklin *et al.*, 2015).

Children with disabilities are often viewed as less credible reporters of violence (Cederborg and Lamb, 2006; Bettenay *et al.*, 2014; Brown and Lewis, 2013; Bottoms, 2003; Henry *et al.*, 2011; Niehaus *et al.*, 2013). A recent study using thirty-two in-depth interviews in Scotland confirms this among police and other professionals (Stalker *et al.*, 2015).

Implicit bias and empathy for caregiver

In addition, past research has found that children with disabilities are less likely to have substantiated reports because of bias/attitudes/lack of training of authorities throughout the process (Manders and Stoneman, 2009). In research on child welfare workers, Cooke and Standen (2002) discovered that workers had a tendency 'not to see' abuse among children with disabilities, in part because of lack of training. The consequences of abuse among children not being recognised as abusive were that these children were not being registered with CPS and therefore not receiving intervention. A sample drawn from a number of serious case reviews in England examined children's developmental needs and identified a number of developmentally harmful behaviours by caregivers in respect of children with disabilities (Brandon *et al.*, 2012; 2008). The increased vulnerability of children with disabilities was becoming well-recognised and was a feature in 12% of these serious case reviews. The risk of harm went unrecognised in these cases, sometimes in cases where the family was presented as loving and cooperative. They discovered that there was a tendency to see the disability more clearly than the child, and this could mean accepting a different and lower standard of parenting for a child with disabilities than would be tolerated for a child without disabilities (e.g. keeping a child shut in a bedroom for long periods for 'safety'). Practitioners were found to be reassured by their 'good' relationship with the parent, but it did not necessarily mean that children were kept safe.

In the vignette study by Manders and Stoneman (2009) described earlier, most CPS workers empathised with parents, which influenced their treatment of the abuse cases. Abuse was often attributed to characteristics of the child's disability and in cases (or hypothetical cases) where the child had a disability they were treated differently even when the abuse was severe (broken bones, concussion, etc.) (Manders and Stoneman, 2009; Rogers *et al.*, 2009).

One of the benefits of agency data is that it often captures cases that are not substantiated. Through asking agency workers about the cases of abuse they have seen, we are able to capture those who have been brought to the attention of authorities (even if not substantiated).

Institutional issues/constraints and resources

Beyond bias and empathy of the individuals involved in the system, there are also systemic issues in terms of being able to support children with disabilities in the child welfare system. Research shows that, when children with disabilities enter the child welfare system, social services are often not prepared to service their needs adequately (Shannon and Tappan, 2011). In an ethnographic study of child welfare workers in the US, researchers found that many case workers do not have proper placement in homes or access to counselling services appropriate for children with disabilities, among other things (ibid.). Research from Scotland found similar results, indicating that the child was often not the focus of the intervention/treatment and that child protection workers were 'muddling through' and not necessarily providing the best care or services for children with disabilities (Taylor *et al.*, 2015b). In addition to empathy for caregivers, caseworkers were also working within a system in which they might have felt that the children, while not in a good circumstance, did not have better alternatives.

When considering how to handle a new case of abuse, social workers may be asking themselves if they have enough people and resources to handle the case. Lack of appropriate services and quality care placements is also a concern for children with disabilities entering the child welfare system (Taylor *et al.*, 2015a). Research on sexual exploitation of children with learning disabilities found that the resources available are very inconsistent and variable across agencies and localities. Moreover, even among places with supports in place for children with disabilities, only 41% of local authorities felt their services were actually meeting the needs of young people with disabilities (Franklin *et al.*, 2015).

Ethical considerations

Keeping children safe and maintaining their privacy are crucial when collecting data on children. This is particularly important when considering a topic such as victimisation, in which there is an ethical necessity to report ongoing threats to children while at the same time wanting to collect information on children and ensure their participation in research. Including children with disabilities and allowing them to engage in research is also an ethical imperative. Research comparing proxy and self-reports indicates that proxy reports (by caregivers) undercount experiences with victimisation (Chan *et al.*, 2014). It is unclear in the literature the extent to which children with disabilities are excluded from research or are replaced with parent/proxy reports because of barriers to inclusion (e.g. access to registered sign language interpreters, materials in braille). Chapter 4 presents case studies that detail the experiences of and challenges faced by researchers in designing research studies inclusive of children with disabilities.

Researchers have long been concerned with the impact of engaging in the research process with children. Surprisingly though, there is limited empirical evidence on the consequences of directly questioning victims, particularly among those with disabilities. A recent article examined the influence of participating in the National Survey of Children's Exposure to Violence (NatSCEV) on children ages 10–17. Overall, researchers found that the vast majority of children were not upset with taking the survey (which included fifty-three victimisation items from the JVQ). In total, 4.5% of the sample reported being upset at all, and just 0.8% were 'pretty/a lot' upset (Finkelhor *et al.*, 2014b). Research of this type needs to be replicated with participants with disabilities, examining if there are any differences in experiences with taking the survey for children with disabilities, and the extent to which children of different types of disability may have varying experiences. (See Chapter 4 for more discussion on this.)

While it is unclear to what extent children with disabilities are impacted by participating in research on victimisation, it is worth discussing methodological ways that we might attenuate any potential negative consequences of participation. One recommendation is to employ longitudinal designs. Longitudinal studies that follow children over time have the advantage of contemporaneous victimisation data, which could serve to reduce risk of re-traumatisation and have the advantage of control for concerns related to the retrospective recall of adverse events (UNICEF, 2012). This may be particularly important for children with specific types of disabilities (e.g. cognitive or developmental disabilities). Longitudinal research would also allow researchers to observe and as a result provide services to help reduce the negative consequences of trauma (from both victimisation and disclosure) and allow researchers to observe how risk for victimisation among children with disabilities varies over time.

Conclusion

We have access to a range of data sources on violence in the lives of children with disabilities. Most of these sources indicate that children with disabilities are at higher risk for victimisation than their peers without disabilities. The extent and exact nature of this relationship remains poorly understood because of methodological and ethical challenges associated with collecting this type of data on a vulnerable and often marginalised population. It is clear that the process of gathering information on victimisation exposure among children with disabilities is complicated and in most if not all stages more challenging for children with disabilities.

After reviewing the stages to inclusion in disability and victimisation data, it is no wonder that children with disabilities are undercounted in research on victimisation. At each stage, children with disabilities face barriers above and beyond those faced by their counterparts without disabilities. We have also seen that these barriers vary by a number of factors including the type of disability. The obstacles faced by children are particularly distressing in that children thought to be at the highest risk, such as those living in institutions or those with 'severe' disabilities, are also least likely to be included in research and in the child welfare system and its reports.

Better data on child victimisation in the lives of children with disabilities could serve to enhance our efforts to protect children at the highest risk and to provide the best possible supports to children who experience victimisation. The inclusion of children with disabilities as participants in research will ideally ultimately contribute to our ability to protect those children at highest risk. It is clear that we do not know about the violence in the lives of many children and that as a child welfare system we are not meeting the needs of those who are identified, specifically children with disabilities.

CHAPTER 3

Making informed consent accessible and engaging for children with disabilities

Audrey Cameron
Associate Tutor (Deaf Education), Moray House School of Education, University of Edinburgh

Introduction

We view participation in research among children with disabilities as essential to understanding the nature and extent of violence in their lives and ultimately to protect those children most vulnerable. Informed consent is a vital part of the research process and as such entails more than merely obtaining a signature on a form. The challenge for researchers is to engage with potential participants and enable them to achieve a level of confidence in making an informed decision about whether or not to contribute to a study. We know that deaf children and children with disabilities are more vulnerable to abuse (Jones *et al.*, 2012; Sullivan & Knutson, 2000; see Chapter 1) and that they face significant barriers when it comes to seeking help (Taylor *et al.*, 2015a). There is an urgent need to include the views of these children in child protection research and to develop a better understanding of what informed consent means to them. For some, this means providing information about the research study in ways that deaf and children with disabilities might more readily understand.

This chapter will offer a brief review of the broader context and reference of a number of studies on the informed consent of children with disabilities. As a researcher and a member of the Deaf community, I have fully explored some issues in relation to d/Deaf children and child protection in the hope of offering broader insights on this topic to other researchers in the field of child protection. Parsons *et al.* (2016) argue that there is a great need to share research methods for gaining informed consent from children. Therefore, in this chapter we suggest a number of practical approaches that researchers may want to consider as they look to enable deaf children and children with disabilities to give their informed consent to participate in research activities. As part of this, the relative merits of using a 'dialogic approach' (Pollard *et al.*, 2009) are considered specifically (but not exclusively) when working with people from the Deaf community.

What is informed consent?

The concept of informed consent in research involving people came from the Nuremberg Code (1948) and later the Declaration of Helsinki (1964) (Weindling, 2001). The Nuremberg Code was established after the trials of the Nazi army, which conducted medical experiments on concentration camp inmates during the Second World War, without their consent (Katz, 1996). This included sterilisation experiments and euthanasia of adults and children with disabilities. The Nuremberg Code states that 'the voluntary consent of the human participant is absolutely essential', i.e. making it clear that participants should give consent and that benefits of research must outweigh the risks. The Declaration of Helsinki was established by the World Medical Association with a set of ethical principles regarding human experimentation.

Looking for ways of enabling potential participants to understand the purpose and aims of the research, and giving informed consent to participate, are now considered a central requirement of any study. This consent needs to be given freely and without coercion, and must be based on a clear understanding of what participation involves. In the UK, the Economic and Social Research Council defines 'freely given informed consent' as:

- giving sufficient and appropriate information about the research, to allow participants to make a meaningful choice about whether or not to take part;
- ensuring that there is no explicit or implicit coercion, so prospective participants can make an informed and free decision on their possible involvement (ESRC, n.d.).

According to the Child Protection Monitoring and Evaluation Reference Group (CP MERG, 2012), informed consent rests on four core principles:

- Consent involves an explicit act, such as a verbal or written agreement;
- Consent can only be given if the participants are informed about, and have an understanding of the research;
- Consent must be given voluntarily and without coercion;
- Consent must be renegotiable so that children may withdraw at any stage of the research process.

Ethical debates on children with disabilities as research participants

There is a growing recognition of the need to involve children in decisions about their lives. The UNCRC emphasises children's rights to freedom of expression, and this includes access to information and expressing their views about matters affecting them (Articles 12 and 13). There are debates on the involvement of children with disabilities in research (see Chapter 5). Different articles from the UNCRC have been cited to make the case that children with disabilities should not be excluded from opportunities to participate in research (Connors and Stalker, 2003; Feldman *et al.*, 2013; Garth and Aroni, 2003; Lewis and Porter, 2004; Loveridge and Meyer, 2010; MacArthur *et al.*, 2007). Article 2 emphasises the principles of non-discrimination. Therefore, denying children with disabilities from participation in research will be discrimination. Article 23 states that children with disabilities have the right to enjoy a full and decent life and to actively participate in the community.

Because of the way our societies are organised, children with disabilities have been found to be more vulnerable to abuse (Jones *et al.*, 2012; Sullivan and Knutson, 2000). Despite the additional vulnerabilities, there is a relative lack of research and we still know very little about the views and experiences of children with disabilities when it comes to child protection. Only a few studies, primarily in high-income countries, have asked children with disabilities directly for their views on the child protection system (see, for example, Taylor *et al.*, 2015a; Jones *et al.*, 2016; Stalker *et al.*, 2010; for an example in LMICs see Uganda case study in Chapter 4, Kuper *et al.*, 2016). If we seek to value the contribution that children and young people with disabilities can bring to our understanding (not just researchers), then we need to find ways to involve children with disabilities in our research.

This principle lies at the core of what we consider to be ethical practice and empowerment.

Cavet and Sloper (2004) were able to demonstrate that children with disabilities can hold and express their views if given a platform in the right environment, and that they value participation in research. Rabiee *et al.* (2005) conclude that 'exclusion of disabled children from research and consultation says more about unsuitability of research and consultation methods and adults not knowing how to relate to them about the limitations on the part of informants' (Rabiee *et al.*, 2005, p. 387). Booth and Booth (1996) also suggest that 'researchers should attend more to their deficiencies than to the limitations of their informants' (p. 67). If no appropriate tools are developed, this group of children will be excluded from research. Examples of appropriate and accessible tools are discussed later in this chapter, and a case study of how these have been applied in research is presented in Chapter 4.

Increased ethical regulation from Research Ethic Committees (REC), Research Ethic Boards (REB) and Institutional Review Boards (IRB) over the past twenty years means that researchers now have less latitude to make decisions about the ways in which informed consent processes are managed, and there are more formal consent procedures to be followed when working with children (Alderson and Morrow, 2006; Miller and Boulton, 2007; Parsons *et al.*, 2016; Wiles *et al.*, 2007). IRB is the terminology used throughout this book when referring to these formal independent institutional or national ethical reviews of research. These are called IRBs in the US and many countries globally and Ethics Review Boards in the UK. This is distinguished from informal expert review and input into study design, analysis and dissemination in the form of Research Advisory Committees (RACs). Additional safeguarding measures are in place to obtain consent from children with disabilities in many EU member states at the national level, including Greece, Ireland and Poland (EU FRA, 2014), which has practical and methodological implications for researchers, and may even discourage them from pursuing research with this population (University of Sheffield, 2015). Despite the increasing scrutiny, there is a need for researchers to take a creative and flexible approach to informed consent that more closely reflects the needs of the children with disabilities they are working with (Parsons *et al.*, 2016; Wiles *et al.*, 2007). In recent years, research teams have been focusing on the concept of informed consent in relation to deaf children and children with disabilities and how best to obtain it (Alderson, 1995; Beresford, 1997; Cocks, 2006; 2008; Connors and Stalker, 2003; Singleton *et al.*, 2014; Ward, 1997; Young and Hunt, 2011; Young and Temple, 2014).

Some research teams have worked with deaf researchers, researchers with disabilities or young people to ensure they were providing accessible information (Connors and Stalker, 2003; Jones, 2004; McKee *et al.*, 2013; Tarleton *et al.*, 2004; Taylor *et al.*, 2015a; Young and Temple, 2014). A two-year qualitative study in Scotland that explored the views and experiences of children with disabilities and their siblings involved two young people with disabilities in the initial design of the study (Connors and Stalker, 2003), and another UK study recruited an advisory group of young people with learning disabilities to provide input on the informed consent forms and interview guide (Franklin *et al.*, 2015; see also Chapter 4). Similarly, the Deaf and Disabled Children Talking about Child Protection (DDTCP) research study in the UK received guidance on the study design and data-collection techniques from members of the study's research advisory group and three young disabled advisors. One of the members of the research team was also Deaf and fluent in British Sign Language (BSL) (Taylor *et al.*, 2015a). These examples show how considering different strategies for making the information available about the research can make it accessible for all children. We need to be aware that children's needs and abilities exist on a spectrum.

'Capacity' to consent

One of the difficulties with the notion of informed consent is that the way it is presented. No matter in what manner/format this is done, it still requires the participants to be able to process or analyse information in a specific way (i.e. to receive the information and familiarise themself with the underlying concepts, and to work through the costs and benefits before deciding on a course of action). As Nind (2008) points out, this can be challenging for those with communication difficulties and learning disabilities, and the question soon becomes one of 'capacity'. Those with memory and/or problem-solving difficulties may also struggle to express their views (in a conventional manner).

If a child can be judged to understand what participation in research will involve (known as 'Gillick competence' – Hunter and Pierscionek, 2007) then parental consent will not be required. Consent from a parent or guardian is necessary in relation to research with children and with adults who lack the capacity to give consent for themselves. Depending on where the research is being carried out, the researchers have to consider the country's rules, regulations and guidelines on obtaining informed consent from the child and their parents: for example, in Europe the child's age limit for obtaining parental consent varies. In some countries such as Ireland, Germany, Greece and Portugal, parental consent is always required for children up to eighteen years old (EU FRA, 2014). This is the same in the US. For other countries such as the UK, Hungary and Finland, parent consent is required up to 15–16 years old. However, if the young person is vulnerable or has a disability, the age limit is increased to eighteen years old. There are no clear regulations about parental consent in France, Spain, Italy, Austria, Slovakia and Denmark.

It is not ethical to ask parents to consent on behalf of the child, and if possible parental consent should be obtained in advance of the child's consent to avoid the situation in which the child has agreed but finds that they are not allowed to participate. Researchers also cannot assume that once they receive parental consent the child will want to participate. However, involving parents or carers can also present additional ethical challenges such as privacy and confidentiality (see Figure 5.4 for Kelly's case study). Parental consent may be waived in some cases to preserve the child's confidentiality – such as if the child was using a service like a sexual health service or a drug treatment agency.

What do we mean by 'capacity'? Capacity requires a degree of autonomy and ability to make decisions. For many children with disabilities, opportunities to learn are restricted or even denied to them (Young and Temple, 2014). When we consent to something, does that mean we will have a full and complete understanding of what we are consenting to, and what the respective implications are for us if we decide to consent or not? Is it a question of satisfying ourselves that we have an 'adequate understanding', and if so shouldn't this be the benchmark? In current practice, capacity to consent to participate in research is often determined by the researcher. It would be beneficial to develop standardised ways to determine capacity to ensure individuals are not excluded from research.

For example, typical consent forms are written in English, yet many deaf people struggle with factual knowledge (commonly referred to as limited fund of information) because they do not have enough access to information in sign language, which impacts on their literacy (Pollard *et al.*, 2009; Young and Hunt, 2011). Language in many informed consent documents requires a high level of English, and this will also cause an impact on people with limited English proficiency and people with learning disabilities (Felzmann *et al.*, 2010). Even the use of sign language interpreters does not guarantee deaf people being able to give informed consent (McKee *et al.*, 2013). In the US, federal regulations governing people-based research stipulate that information should be accessible and comprehensible to all deaf people in their preferred language (McKee *et al.*, 2013). Sudore *et al.* (2006) state that informed consent should be delivered in the participant's preferred language, regardless of their proficiency in English, to maximise the likelihood that consent information will be understood.

Potential approaches to obtaining consent from children with disabilities

Consent as a process

Obtaining consent throughout the research process, rather than just once at the start of the study, has been highlighted as the most ethical type of consent process as it gives the child or young person full control at every stage. Being given the options of choosing whether to proceed or withdraw without any consequences can also reduce anxiety related to participating (CP MERG, 2012; Parsons *et al.*, 2016). Providing multiple opportunities to revisit consent may also be important for young people with different types of disabilities, where the timing or sequencing of events may not be remembered (Knox *et al.*, 2000; Rodgers, 1999; Wilson *et al.*, 2010).

This method has been widely discussed and used in research with children, including those with disabilities. In practice, this involves providing the child with adequate and accessible information about what participation means and watching for signs of refusal in the child throughout the interview (Cocks, 2006; Kelly, 2007). Two research studies also gave participants the option to meet the interviewer on two occasions – to discuss the study and access requirements in the first session before meeting again to speak about their views and experiences of their disability and child protection system respectively (Connors and Stalker, 2007; Taylor *et al.,* 2015a). In the latter research, most participants were prepared to discuss the study with the interviewer in the first meeting after giving informed consent. This could be due to having full access to the information beforehand, and being able to have a discussion with the interviewer before giving consent (Taylor *et al.,* 2015a). This method can be a way to help ensure that participants know and understand the purpose of the research (Cree *et al.,* 2002; NIDCD, 1999) and has been suggested to be an inclusive and appropriate way to obtain consent from all children, irrespective of disability (Cocks, 2006).

Figure 3.1: Recording consent

Obtaining written consent from research participants is typically used by researchers to protect not only themselves but also the participant, as it is seen as an active form of 'opting-in' to the research (Wiles et al., 2005, p. 16). When researching sensitive topics, however, verbal instead of written consent is often used to protect confidentiality and hence avoid a record linking the participant to the research study (CP MERG, 2012; Wiles et al., 2007). Signing consent forms can also be problematic for those with language or communication difficulties, and can also 'formalise' the research process, which has been suggested could be 'off-putting' for some (Wiles et al., 2005, p. 17). All of these issues have been highlighted as potential challenges for research specifically with individuals with disabilities, and when studying sensitive topics such as violence. A number of studies have developed alternative methods of obtaining consent, including tape-recorded consent or holding up red or green cards to indicate positive or negative responses (see, for example, Parsons et al., 2016). In the DDTCP study in the UK, confidentiality was maintained by asking participants to tick boxes on the consent form to confirm that they were happy to participate and whether they were comfortable with the interview being recorded (Taylor et al, 2015a). This method was also preferred for participants who may have difficulty in writing, and verbal and signed consent was recorded at the interviews in video or audio (Taylor et al, 2015a). Utilising alternate methods of recording consent has the potential to mitigate important issues such as language barriers and confidentiality and should be carefully considered when designing research with children with disabilities.

A dialogic approach

Parsons *et al.* (2016) reveal that one of the main findings from their interviews with thirty-two social science researchers in the UK was 'the importance of context, sensitivity and relationships for negotiating consent for research participation with children and other vulnerable groups' (Parsons *et al.*, 2016, p. 138). This was also confirmed by Crow *et al.* (2006), Nind (2008) and Young and Temple (2014). A dialogic approach is one example of how measures to obtain consent can be adapted in order to be more appropriate for the deaf population. First described by Pollard *et al.* (2009; 2014), a dialogic approach to consent involves showing Deaf sign language users a video of a signed conversation between two sign language users about the meaning of informed consent. Findings suggested this is a more culturally appropriate way to ensure that Deaf sign language users understand the study's information, and can genuinely give their informed consent. Users reported that the adapted product was more relevant, engaging and effective for deaf audiences (Pollard *et al.*, 2009). Watching a film of two Deaf people discussing the research study will assure some deaf participants who may be unwilling to ask questions about the consent form during the interview, because they are concerned that they do not have the background to understand the answer (NIDCD, 1999; Pollard *et al.*, 2009; Young and Temple, 2014).

This approach also proved invaluable when recruiting children and adults with disabilities for a study conducted in the UK about child protection (Taylor *et al.*, 2015a). The research team adopted Pollard's approach and produced a film showing two Deaf people – the researcher and a young actress acting as a participant – discussing, in BSL, the consent form and the participation information sheet. The BSL video clip also had a voice-over narrative to enable any participant to have access to the dialogic film. During the interviews, the Deaf participants confirmed that they found this dialogic method useful to help them to prepare for the interview (Taylor *et al.*, 2015a). Subtitled videos also made these films accessible for deaf people who do not sign. This 'dialogic approach' is a potentially useful avenue to explore for future child protection research, including in LMICs.

Accessible material

Accessibility is imperative when obtaining free and informed consent (Alderson, 2004; Connors and Stalker, 2003). This is also important in order to avoid overwhelming potential participants with information.

In this context, accessibility involves the layout, colour, font, type of language used and the inclusion of images on the study information sheets. The rest of this chapter will outline practical ways to create accessible information for different needs.

Simple wording of text

It is important to review the actual text of an information sheet and how this is constructed and presented, because it may have an impact on the ability of some children to access it effectively. Long and complicated sentences may be difficult for the reader to understand. Some guidelines for simplifying text include:

- write in short simple sentences (no longer than 15–20 words);
- be conscious of where sentences begin on the page, as starting a new sentence at the end of a line makes it harder to follow;
- try to call the readers 'you', imagining they are sitting opposite you and you are talking to them directly;
- give instructions clearly. Avoid long sentences of explanation;
- use lists where appropriate: lists are excellent for splitting information up (Ranalidi and Nisbet, 2010).

Use of pictures and symbols

Pictorial and simply worded documents can be created for those with communication difficulties or learning disabilities. Pictures are always useful to support text, making the meaning clearer and easier to understand. They provide a visual representation of a concept and act as 'concrete' points of reference, pinning language down and if necessary helping to refocus attention on a particular idea.

Research and practical experience have shown that all children respond well to graphic support for written and spoken language, whether or not they have particular difficulties with language and/ or reading (Alderson, 2004; Ranalidi and Nisbet, 2010; Connors and Stalker, 2003; Kelly, 2007; Wiles *et al.*, 2007). For those who have any kind of additional support needs (e.g. English as a second or additional language, learning difficulties, speech language and communication impairments, or literacy difficulties), graphic support is an essential lifeline, giving access to the curriculum and to everyday information in the community.

Symbol sets and symbol software have been developed in response to this need, providing a comprehensive collection of images specially designed with an internal logic and coherence. These images share a consistent 'look' and size/shape, which give greater support than 'random' clip art, can be shared throughout an establishment or across the community as a 'shared language', and are more practical to use.

Mayer Johnston Picture Communication Symbols (PCS)

PCS symbols (also known as Boardmaker™ Symbols) are commonly used as 'single' images to illustrate a general concept and/or to stimulate and support discussion and explanation (available from URL: http://uk.mayer-johnson.com/default.aspx; accessed 27 April 2016). These symbols are widely used across the UK, in both schools and adult services, by children with various types of communication disorders. PCS comprises a vocabulary of approximately 9,000 symbols. The DDTCP research study pictorial information sheet was created with PCS symbols (Taylor *et al.*, 2015a).

Widgit™ symbols

Pictorial consent can also be created using Widgit™ symbols from the Widgit™ software (available from URL: www.widgit.com/about-symbols/best-practice/index.htm; accessed 27 April 2016). It is also known as Communicate in Print (part of the 'Communicate' range of software, including SymWriter). Widgit™ is a British company that specialises in the use of symbols to support inclusion. Widgit™ symbols are designed to support access to the curriculum in UK schools and in particular to assist access to text and literacy development. They are sometimes therefore used almost as a 'word for word' translation of connected text.

Both of the above systems include symbols particularly relevant to sex education/sexuality/sexual abuse, although these may need to be purchased and installed separately. They are not part of the main 'classic' symbol systems. Research teams have employed these symbol systems when creating information sheets and consent forms (Cocks, 2006; Mitchell and Sloper, 2011).

Talking Mats™

These can be used as a communication tool when discussing face to face with a potential participant about the research project (Rabiee *et al.*, 2005). Talking Mats™ provide textured mats with cards showing the symbols. This resource was developed by a team of speech and language therapists to help people overcome communication difficulties, and to give them their say by placing the communication symbols on a mat to enable people to listen to them (e.g. people with a learning disability or who suffered from stroke, dementia, etc.). At the top of the mat, there are special symbols showing what you might be feeling. Cards can be placed under a specific symbol at the top to indicate how you are feeling.

This tool is frequently used by clinical practitioners, carers and support workers in a wide range of health, social work, residential and education settings. It can be very useful when asking for the views of young children with communication difficulties. Talking Mats™ also have an App that can be used with iPad, Android or personal computer.

Accessible material for people with visual impairment

An information sheet and consent form with large text (16 point) in Arial font should be provided for people with visual impairment or limited vision. They should also be given an option of an electronic copy of the documents to allow them to magnify or amend the documents to their preferred font and size on their computers.

The Royal National Institute of the Blind (RNIB, n.d.) in the UK recommends the following:

- regular print of the text is to be at 10 or 12 point;
- large print is to be significantly bigger – 16 point or higher – and this may be large enough for people who have some useful sight, but struggle to read regular print;
- giant print is to be larger than 18-point size.

RNIB also states that it is important to check with the potential participants with visual impairment to discover what size of font they are comfortable reading. RNIB has produced a specialist font that is legible to people with limited vision – Tiresias. This font is designed to have characters that are easy to distinguish from each other. (It can be downloaded for free from URL: www.fontsquirrel.com/fonts/

Tiresias-Infofont; accessed 31 January 2017.) Tiresias is actually a figure from Greek mythology, a blind prophet from Thebes.

Some people may prefer an audio recording of the research material. This can be uploaded to a research project webpage along with the information sheets and consent forms.

Sign language video clips for deaf people

BSL is a visual-gestural language that is the first or preferred language of many deaf people and some deaf/blind people living in the UK (Brennan, 1990). Contrary to common belief, it is not a manual version of English: the language has its own grammar and syntax differing from English (Sutton-Spence and Woll, 1999) and signs are created by combining hand shapes with locations and movement. Different countries around the world have their own sign language: for example, American Sign Language (ASL) for the US; Libras for Brazil; Langue des Signes Française (LSF) for France; and Auslan for Australia.

Consent forms are usually written in ways that are inaccessible for people whose second language is English. Many deaf people struggle to understand spoken English and may lack proficiency in written English (McKee *et al.*, 2013). It is a common practice that research teams working with Deaf people create video clips of sign language to explain the research in their preferred language, because it is culturally and linguistically appropriate and because it will ensure good processes of consent (McKee *et al.*, 2013; NIDCD, 1999: Pollard *et al.*, 2009; Singleton *et al.*, 2014; Taylor *et al.*, 2015a; Young and Hunt, 2011, Young and Temple, 2014).

Similarly, as discussed earlier, a dialogic approach can be employed by showing Deaf participants a video of a signed conversation between sign language users about consent. This has been used among adults (Pollard *et al.*, 2009; 2014) and children, specifically on child protection (Taylor *et al.*, 2015a) and has been shown to be an effective adaptation to elicit free and informed consent. This approach might be useful for anyone.

Conclusion

This chapter has provided a number of practical suggestions for researchers to consider when they are looking to work with children with disabilities in their research activities. Crucially, the process of informed consent should be made accessible to all participants, and there are a number of ways to accomplish this, all of which require careful planning and an understanding of the study population. This can be best achieved by involving children and young people with disabilities in all phases of the research or by using researchers with disabilities. The benefits of adopting a dialogic approach (Pollard *et al.*, 2009) to informed consent is a potentially important area to develop further in research on violence against children with disabilities.

CHAPTER 4

The challenges and promising practices for researching violence against children with disabilities: Case studies from around the world

Patricia Lannen[1] *and Tabitha Casey*[2]

1 Program Director Child Protection, UBS Optimus Foundation, Zurich
2 Project Manager for the Safe Inclusive Schools Network, Moray House School of Education, University of Edinburgh

Introduction

In this chapter, we introduce a range of examples of research on violence against children with disabilities from different parts of the world. While Chapter 2 provides an overview of data sources and challenges associated with collecting data on violence against children with disabilities, this chapter builds a timely summary of lessons learnt and good practices. It also highlights methodological and research gaps in need of further attention by drawing on published works as well as interviews with the researchers who conducted the studies. The chapter includes studies – some recently completed, some still ongoing – from the US, the UK, Switzerland, Hong Kong, Burundi and Uganda. They were chosen to represent a variety of different methodologies, including longitudinal studies and evaluations of prevention programmes, as well as studies focused on experiences of victims with the support they received.

Drawing on the current knowledge and recent experience of researchers, we delve into issues related to planning processes, implementation challenges, lessons learnt and perhaps most illuminating what the researchers would recommend for future research efforts. Findings are presented by the ethical and methodological issues identified by the researchers, and they aim to provide practical examples of how different researchers have dealt with some of the key challenges identified in previous chapters. More detailed descriptions of the research studies can be found in the appendix.

Benefits and risks of research on a sensitive topic with a vulnerable population

When a study is designed to conduct interviews with child victims of violence, there is often a valid concern that participation may cause harm through re-traumatisation (Morris *et al.*, 2012). From the interviews with the researchers it became clear that the ethical concerns around the potential harms of research on the participating individuals increase significantly with children with disabilities, particularly when it is unknown how an individual understands and processes potentially distressing information. This reflects the importance of the discussion around 'Ethical considerations' from Chapter 2 as well as reflections on '"Capacity" to consent' elaborated on in Chapter 3.

However, the UK case study, which explored the service support needs of young people with learning disabilities who experienced or were at risk of experiencing child sexual exploitation (CSE) , found that many participants were eager to share their experiences of CSE, even though they were not asked about this (Franklin *et al.*, 2015). As discussed in Chapter 2, ddditional research could examine whether the concern about the presumed harm of participation in such studies is in fact true, or whether this is based on a false assumption.

Issues around informed consent

Ethical considerations around obtaining informed consent were highlighted by most researchers as an issue requiring careful planning and flexibility. Some of the case studies revealed that for ethical reasons some of the individuals with the most 'severe' disabilities were excluded from being interviewed as part of the research. While Article 12 of the UNCRC (United Nations General Assembly, 1989) emphasises the right to participation, ethical considerations led the researchers to prioritise the protection of these children over participation. (See Chapter 1 for a more detailed discussion on participation and protection, Chapter 2 for challenges to collecting data from children with 'severe' disabilities and Chapter 3 for a more detailed discussion on consent).

An example of this can be seen in the Burundi case study (Lee *et al.*, 2016; Pittaway *et al.*, in prep.), an evaluation of Handicap International's pilot implementation of the Ubuntu Care Project in Burundi, Kenya and Rwanda. The project aims to reduce sexual violence against children, especially those with disabilities, by addressing the problem on an individual, community and national level. It empowers children to become key actors in their own protection while supporting other stakeholders (especially families) to create a safe protective environment. The Ubuntu project in Burundi is currently being evaluated in partnership with researchers from the University of New South Wales. The study included children with physical and sensory disabilities (such as hearing impairment, visual impairment, cerebral palsy), as well as intellectual disabilities. There was a significant ethical concern about the inclusion of children with intellectual disabilities when it was questionable whether the child was able to understand what they were agreeing to participate in. When children's 'severe' intellectual disabilities prevented them from understanding what was happening in the research, they were taken aside and offered alternative activities, based on the belief that if the 'implementer' felt the child could not understand what was going on it was not truly participatory. These children were therefore excluded from the research, despite the concern that evidence suggests that children with the most 'severe' forms of cognitive development are at the highest risk of abuse (Hershkowitz *et al.*, 2007). Nonetheless, it was still possible to access some information related to these children through the participation of their relatives in the population targeted by the evaluation. Furthermore, there is currently no evidence about how to reduce potential researcher bias in making these decisions, and this area – inclusion and exclusion of participants with disabilities – requires further attention.

In Chapter 3, we discussed how 'capacity to consent' relates to the decision of whether parental or child consent is sought and how differences between parental and child consent can be reconciled. In the case study of Burundi (Lee *et al.*, 2016; Pittaway *et al.*, in prep.), parent consent was sought first, then consent was reconfirmed with the children, with opportunities to discontinue participation at any point in the process. A child-friendly version of the consent form was created, under the guidance of the research team in order to make sure that despite simplification of the content of the form the message was not altered. The project team went through the consent form with each child and explained that even if they decided not to participate in the research they would still have access to project activities.

Other case studies did not encounter the same challenges around consent. In the UK case study on CSE services (Franklin *et al.*, 2015), verbal and written consent was obtained from all participants, and also from a parent or carer if the participant was under the age of sixteen. The research, conducted in partnership with Barnardo's and The Children's Society (two leading children's charities that run most of the CSE services in the UK) as well as with the British Institute of Learning Disabilities, did not have issues obtaining parental consent, which the researchers attributed to the well-established relationships the CSE services maintained with the families. The researchers spent time with participants before, during and after the research process to ensure that they understood what the research entailed, that they could stop at any time, and that they could withdraw their data for a certain time period after the research concluded.

The case of the UK study (Franklin *et al.*, 2015) highlights the important role of gatekeepers and services in the process of recruiting and facilitating individuals to take part in research studies. Collaborating with organisations that have already established relationships and trust with potential research participants and their guardians might prove to be crucial for research success.

Planning the research

There were many methodological issues that were considered by researchers in the planning stage of research. The UK researchers (Franklin *et al.*, 2015) highlighted the importance of maintaining flexibility in this stage. Access to the target population was limited as the CSE services through which recruitment was conducted focus on crisis management, and they only provide services to young people for a short space of time following their experience of CSE. This meant that the researchers needed to be adaptable to the availability of participants, which had both time and budgetary implications. While it is necessary to be flexible in order to recruit participants and meet the target sample size, it may also create selection bias. This topic is reviewed in more detail in Chapter 2. This was also mentioned by researchers working in low-resource settings but for different reasons. In the Burundi case study (Lee *et al.*, 2016; Pittaway *et al.*, in prep.), researchers highlighted the need for careful planning in relation to budgeting and logistics to find a safe place for all to come together, and to account for participants who may need to travel long distances to the study site and/or stay overnight. This was seen as an absolute prerequisite before the start of any activities in order to make sure that the accommodation was accessible. Accessibility was defined in terms of funds available for safe transport, as well as physical accessibility for children with disabilities and the child protection measures in place for transport to the interview site.

Another key finding of these case studies was the importance of involving research expertise from both fields – disability and violence – so that challenges can be identified and solved jointly. In Uganda (Devries *et al.*, 2014), where researchers conducted an evaluation of Raising Voices' school-based violence-prevention programme 'Good School Toolkit', researchers felt this was crucial to the success of the project. In the UK (Franklin *et al.*, 2015), the team had extensive training in child protection, and also had experience working with children with disabilities. The researchers felt it was essential to have specialised skills in both areas to be confident in identifying safeguarding concerns; it was also beneficial in the planning stage. In Burundi (Lee *et al.*, 2016; Pittaway *et al.*, in prep.), the researchers felt that having Handicap International staff trained in child protection as well as the researchers' background as former social workers were key to the success of the study.

As the discourse related to 'participation' versus 'protection' has unfolded and shifted from research 'on' children to research 'with' children (Gilligan, 2015), some studies have found innovative ways to encourage youth participation and include children and adolescents as a way to ensure ethical research. An excellent example of making use of youth participation in research is the UK case study (Franklin *et al.*, 2015). The expertise they made sure to have available throughout the process made this study unique. It had two advisory groups, which consulted on aspects of the study throughout: one was a professional reference group of practitioners and academics; and the other comprised five young people with learning disabilities who had experienced CSE. The members of the latter were recruited from two services, had actively participated together as part of other consultation groups, and were therefore already knowledgeable about ethical considerations around confidentiality and anonymity. They had not participated in research projects, however, so the researchers made sure they understood the process and what would be expected of them. The interview schedule, informed consent forms and information sheets were developed with the input of this advisory group. After data collection, the group then met for a second time to discuss the findings and recommendations, specifically how well they felt the recommendations reflected the needs of young people with learning disabilities. The researchers highlighted the value of their input, particularly around appropriate wording and structuring the guide. Involving young people with learning disabilities in an advisory capacity was recommended for future work, though researchers stress the importance of investing enough time to ensure appropriate support mechanisms are in place, and to ensure young people feel empowered in their role.

In addition, it was reported to be beneficial to have the implementing organisation closely involved throughout the research to help facilitate, to train staff on how to interact with study participants, and to plan in time to break the ice. In Burundi, the researchers allowed time for icebreaker activities for everyone, including staff and researchers to become comfortable with some of the more sensitive topics including disability and abuse. In addition, researchers emphasised the importance of collaborating with disabled persons organisations when planning research with children with disabilities, and to include the children themselves in this process. Similar to the experience of the UK study related to recruitment and consent discussed earlier, the implementing organisation that had already gained the trust of the participants and had specific expertise in how to connect with the individuals participating in the research was crucial for research success.

Another important component in designing this type of research is to consider children's evolving capacity and that the impact of exposure to violence on a child with a disability might be related to the age of the child and how the child is able to process information. A child that is being teased for a disability at age five might respond very differently to a child in the same situation at age fifteen, hence coping and impact of a situation is likely to be age-specific. We often talk about children as one group, when age and gender are very important. Particularly in the Uganda study (Devries et al., 2014) there was a perceived need to understand how evolving capacity and resiliency influence the impact of violence on the lives of children with disabilities. Designing research that captures this or is able to extrapolate relevant information will be essential. In addition, improving availability of evidence on resiliency and how children cope with disability and violence were noted as key to informing future programming.

Methodological adjustments and instrument design

Several studies were described where the methodology was adjusted to allow children with disabilities to take part in the research. Adjustments naturally varied for the type of disability, each with different challenges that needed to be considered carefully. For example, in the Burundi case study (Lee *et al.*, 2016; Pittaway *et al.*, in prep.) means were put in place to facilitate communication depending on the child's disability with the help of adaptations and/or translators. In another related study in Uganda (Kuper *et al.*, 2016), the issue of participant safety and confidentiality was considered when choosing a sign language interpreter for deaf children, for example, in order for the child to be able to trust that anything shared is safe with the sign language interpreter. Preparations and trainings were also held on how to interview children with intellectual disabilities and make sure children understood the questions.

In the UK case study (Franklin *et al.*, 2015), the project worker who liaised with the participant provided additional information to the researchers before the interview, with the young person's permission. The project worker gave advice on support needs as well as information on the individual's situation. They were also asked for their thoughts on the suitability of the interview instrument for each individual, another example of how gatekeepers and services can proactively be included to optimise the research process.

Another methodological issue that arose was how to design accessible study instruments while ensuring that the item's purpose or an explanation remains the same even if simplified. For qualitative research in the UK, the interview guide drew on existing work in this area (Stalker, 2013; Taylor *et al.*, 2015a) and was organised by theme, as suggested by the study's advisory groups. The interviews with young people with learning disabilities who had experienced or were at risk of CSE focused on five themes:

- the reason for referral to a CSE service and the information they had received during the referral process;

- the support they received at the service, and their opinion about what worked and what did not;
- the impact or outcomes they experienced from using the CSE service;
- their opinions on how the support could have been improved; and
- any gaps they identified in support provision (including other services such as education and social care) (see Franklin *et al.*, 2015, pp. 16–17).

Using a thematic approach was thought to allow participants to answer whichever questions they felt comfortable with, and to foster a relaxed and accessible environment. Although researchers planned to adapt the guide to meet more complex needs, this was ultimately not necessary for this project. Researchers hypothesised this could be because children with more 'severe' disabilities were not being identified as requiring CSE services, possibly because of increased social isolation or misconceptions that they were not at risk of or experiencing CSE.

Other researchers opted to reduce the number of items used to assess violence. The questionnaire for the Hong Kong case study, a large survey on violence victimisation among school-aged children, contained twelve questions on child maltreatment (psychological violence, corporal punishment and physical violence), parental interpersonal violence and in-law conflict between parents and grandparents. A follow-up survey using a different questionnaire based on the Abuse Assessment Screen (Tiwari *et al.*, 2007) included only five items to assess interpersonal violence from the victim's perspective. The purpose of using fewer questions in this study, instead of other detailed and validated scales, was to minimise respondent burden. While this was considered to be a feasible way to assess violence with this population and a necessary adjustment in order not to overburden participants, there was a concern of potential underreporting. Research indicates that fewer items might affect prevalence rates, and this may be particularly important when measuring sexual violence (Stoltenborgh *et al.*, 2011; Fang *et al.*, 2015). It might therefore be necessary to consider this when choosing or adapting measurements when working with this group of children (see Chapter 1 for a more detailed discussion on how survey design can affect prevalence rates of violence against children).

Defining and measuring disability

Several discussions and considerations were noted around how to define, categorise and operationalise disability, specifically whether to include categories such as learning disabilities, memory problems, concentration difficulties and emotional and behavioural problems. This in turn may have an impact on how disability is assessed, as some might not be detected in self-report, but may require additional sources of information such as psychometric testing. Other topics related to measuring disability came up regarding time-consistency of disability and the finding that some disabilities might change over time (e.g. they might arise as a result of an accident; some might be treatable or others may be detected only as the child grows older). See Chapter 2 for a more comprehensive discussion on this topic.

Some studies avoided the issue of having to define and measure disability as part of the research themselves, by utilising a specific sampling frame. In the Hong Kong case study (Chan *et al.*, 2014), children with disabilities in the study were granted special education services by the Hong Kong Education Bureau, and enrolled in regular schools. Disabilities included visual impairment, hearing impairment, physical disability and intellectual disability. Allocation of 'disability' was done by the schools, and no items on disability were included in the questionnaire.

The Longitudinal Studies on Child Abuse and Neglect (LONGSCAN) (Knight *et al.*, 2000), is a group of research studies on child maltreatment among a cohort of high-risk children; it does not specifically focus on disability. Researchers reported that they had many discussions around how to measure health status during the planning stage: disability was not considered as a specific factor that may make children more vulnerable to abuse and neglect, but rather an aspect of individual health status. LONGSCAN researchers reported that to date they had not analysed these disability measurements. In fact, as part of the search for suitable case studies for this chapter many researchers said that while they recognise, particularly in hindsight, that disability is an important risk factor for violence they reported not necessarily prioritising it. This was mostly either because of lack of expertise in the team or because focusing the research on violence against children more broadly was considered already a complex endeavour in itself.

The UK case study (Franklin *et al.*, 2015) sought to study CSE specifically among young people with learning disabilities, which were defined as a chronic impairment in intelligence and social functioning beginning in childhood. In addition to learning disabilities, a number of participants were described as having autism spectrum conditions, emotional and behavioural difficulties and mental health needs, among other conditions. Establishing inclusion criteria was discussed extensively among all research partners. Ultimately, it was decided not to adhere to a strict definition of learning disability, but rather be guided by the social model of disability, which moves the focus of disability from an individual impairment to societal barriers that in effect 'disable' (UPIAS, 1975). For this study, this meant that the project workers at the CSE services guided the selection of young people by identifying those they believed to have learning barriers. The young people were fully aware they had been put forward for the study because their project workers knew they had struggled or were struggling at school, were having difficulty in comprehending the work they were doing at the CSE service (e.g. around understanding CSE or learning how to keep safe) or that they were being assessed for the first time for a variety of impairments – not only learning disabilities but also attention deficit hyperactivity disorder (ADHD) or autism spectrum. Few participants self-identified as having learning disabilities, but all spoke about difficulties they had in school such as struggling to keep up. Researchers reported that applying a broader approach allowed them to access a group of young people who may not have an official diagnosis of learning disability, but still faced barriers to learning.

As discussed in Chapter 2, researchers are still debating how to best operationalise and measure disability and victimisation. The researchers in the Uganda case study (Devries *et al.*, 2014) emphasised the importance of using standardised approaches to measure disability in order to ensure comparability and to ensure that the measures are a validated way of measuring disability that provide an accurate prevalence. Using the Washington Group 'Short set of questions' (CDC, 2015), they measured disability in the domains of sight, hearing, mobility, speech and whether or not students had epilepsy by asking six questions each with multiple response options. As mentioned in Chapter 2, this tool focuses on how an individual functions within their environment, asking about difficulties walking or climbing steps, difficulties remembering or concentrating, difficulties with communication such as understanding or being understood, etc. The questions are therefore context specific and provide information on how well people are doing in their particular circumstances, rather than a blanket level for all.

In addition, researchers of the Uganda study (Devries *et al.*, 2014) stated that children with an inability to concentrate, memory issues or other learning disabilities should be included, particularly when working in a school setting. This seems particularly important to consider when working with children in low-resource settings, as this might be a heightened concern in areas of prevalent nutritional deficiencies in some poverty-stricken regions. There might be a need to distinguish between acute and long-term disability as different conditions can be treated or change over time. In case of nutritional deficit, symptoms can change when nutritional status improves. Identifying the specific type of impairment was also deemed important, as this would have a key influence on the vulnerability to violence and difficulty in accessing services. This points towards the importance of repeat measures over time to identify those most at risk.

This was done in the Zurich Project on the Social Development of Children in Zurich (z-proso), an ongoing combined longitudinal and intervention study, which has been conducted in Switzerland since 2004 (ETHzürich, n.d.). This showed the value of multi-informant assessment of disability, as a higher correlation of disability between multiple informants might indicate an increased risk of exposure to violence, as well as an increased risk for anxiety and depression. Previously unpublished findings from this study elicited through the interviews conducted for this book (for details see Appendix) found that the correlations of disability measures at age seven (assessed by the mother) with disability measures at age fifteen (self-report) were extremely low or neared zero. However, self-reported bullying victimisation at age fifteen was highest if both informants report a disability. Teacher-assessed internalising symptoms (anxiety and depression) at age fifteen were highest when both informants agreed on presence of disability. In addition, internalising symptoms were also elevated if only the mother reported a disability when the child was aged seven. On the contrary, measure of disability assessed by the mother at child age seven did not predict serious violent victimisation reported by the adolescent at age fifteen. In contrast, self-reported violent victimisation was predicted by concurrent self-reported disability. Hence, the most reliable way to identify those children at risk of violence and mental health issues was when multiple informants agree on disability.

In addition, a few considerations related to these findings could be useful to inform further research:

- Primary caregivers may not have wanted to report emotionally difficult problems for their child, or adolescents may not want to admit to disabilities if they see them as stigmatising.
- The findings could also indicate differences in knowledge. At age seven, potential disabilities such as cognitive disabilities, hearing problems or visual problems may not yet have been known to mothers and were detected only during primary school years.
- Another possibility is that there is actual change over time, which supports the notion that disability should not necessarily always be seen as a time-invariant phenomenon (Roberts *et al.*, 2010). Disabilities such as hearing disabilities or sight disabilities can be treated, they can simply disappear during development, they can emerge at a later stage, or they can be a side effect of environmental events such as accidents.

As mentioned above, these are preliminary findings and warrant a more in-depth analysis. However, the results further point to the importance of repeating data collection of disability over time and, for example, thinking about the relationship between disability and victimisation as – potentially – a reciprocal process. In addition, they further underline the importance of multi-informant measures.

Referral and response system

To have a strong referral and response system to deal competently with any disclosed cases is often a challenge, and to have staff available that are at the same time experienced to support children with disabilities specifically can proof difficult. Nonetheless, this was determined to be essential by many researchers, including the UK (CSE; Franklin *et al.*, 2015) and Burundi (Lee *et al*, 2016; Pittaway *et al.*, in prep.) case studies. It was also one of the key pillars of the research as perceived by the Ugandan team (Devries *et al.*, 2014). A locally active child protection organisation was employed for the time as a referral partner. Tasking an organisation specialised in child protection to take on this role for the duration of the research could potentially be used in other low-resource settings where no referral and response system exists. The researchers perceived that the referral system instilled confidence in all members of the study team to be able to conduct the research on this difficult topic. However, a related study with Plan International on access to child protection for children with disabilities revealed a lack of training of staff in the child protection system on disability, which was perceived to be a major problem (Kuper *et al.*, 2016). This meant that they might not be able to communicate with children with disabilities (e.g. with intellectual or communication impairment) or might have negative attitudes and beliefs about children with disabilities. This underlines some of the findings discussed in Chapter 2 (see 'Training of potential reporters') and could be overcome by making sure that disability sensitisation training is provided to these staff.

Conclusion

By interviewing the researchers of these studies, we have been able to present key insights not available elsewhere. Overall, the interviews conducted to write this chapter confirmed considerable consensus among researchers on the importance of placing greater focus on addressing violence against children with disabilities.

A key learning from the lengthy process of identifying suitable case studies was that, despite or maybe because of the complexity, few studies documented methodological and ethical decisions in detail and generally did not record considerations that went into making these important decisions. When attempting to retrieve this information in personal communication, an additional challenge was that the staff collecting data were generally more junior and employed on temporary contracts, meaning they had often left their positions by the time the interviews were conducted; thus it was difficult or impossible to retrieve information *ex post facto*, and the field knowledge was lost. This makes this learning even more crucial to ensure important lessons about this kind of research are not lost.

However, by interviewing researchers who have specific experience in this field, we have presented new and important lessons that can be drawn upon in future research. Some of the main findings from the research that was explored include: the need to involve specific research expertise both on disability as well as on violence, to tackle a highly complex and ethically challenging issue; the importance of close collaboration with implementers to create trust; the reason to have a solid referral and response system in place that is competent to deal with victims with disability; the potential of measuring disability by multiple informants and repeatedly over time; and the need to understand how to assess the potential ethical risks of research better. Overall, the discussions highlighted the importance of starting to compile good systematic practices for future research so that we can build momentum and increase the evidence base on this complex but important topic.

CHAPTER 5

Ethical and child protection recommendations for researching, documenting and monitoring violence against children with disabilities

Deborah Fry
Lecturer in Child Protection, Moray House School of Education, University of Edinburgh

Introduction

This chapter presents ten key interrelated ethical and protection issues based on findings throughout the chapters of this book that apply specifically to the study of child protection and disability. Key considerations include the need to balance respondents' right to participation in research while maintaining the highest level of ethical standards and ensuring the benefits to respondents or communities of documenting violence against children with disabilities are greater than the risks to respondents and communities. Comprehensive training covering the background of child protection and disability, the study protocol, safeguarding and referral pathways, safety for researchers as well as quality assurance of the data should be provided for all members of the research team including interpreters. Finally, research should also be conducted in such a way so as to maximise benefit to survivors of violence, participants and the community.

These key issues complement and add to existing professional and ethical guidelines applying to research with children or research on sensitive issues such as violence. As such these key areas should not be viewed as all-inclusive or as a stand-alone guide for information gathering about violence against children with disabilities but as a series of key issues to consider based on lessons learnt through the case study examples in Chapter 4 and the increasing learning in this field of research as presented throughout this book.

Figure 5.1: Key ethical guidelines.

Several ethical guideline documents exist for conducting research with children, research on violence against children or research with populations affected by violence. To date, no comprehensive guidelines exist for researching violence against children with disabilities. This chapter builds on these key ethical documents while highlighting the issues unique to research in the area of child protection and disability

○ Ethical Research Involving Children (ERIC) guidelines and website (Graham et al., 2013; www.childethics.com, accessed 31 January 2017). ERIC aims to assist researchers and the research community to understand, plan and conduct ethical research involving children and young people in any geographical, social, cultural or methodological context. It provides an ethical charter as well as a comprehensive ethical guidance document and practical case studies.

○ Ethical principles, dilemmas and risks in collecting data on violence against children. This document represents a comprehensive literature review from the Child Protection Monitoring and Evaluation Reference Group (CP MERG), a global forum for collaboration, coordination and shared learning on child protection monitoring, evaluation and research with representatives from key international child protection organisations as well as academics (CP MERG, 2012; www.cpmerg.org, accessed 31 January 2017).

○ Ethical considerations for the collection, analysis and publication of child maltreatment data. These guidelines were published by the International Society for the Prevention of Child Abuse and Neglect (ISPCAN) in 2016 and provide practical suggestions to researchers for collecting, analysing and publishing child protection data (ISPCAN, 2016; www.ispcan.org, accessed 31 January 2017).

○ World Health Organization (WHO) ethical and safety recommendations for researching, documenting and monitoring sexual violence in emergencies. These guidelines provide comprehensive information to researchers on designing, collecting, analysing and disseminating research related to sexual violence in emergency settings, defined as situations of armed conflict or natural disaster, often involving the displacement of populations, sometimes as refugees, other times as internally displaced people and includes the period of instability which often leads up to an acute crisis and after resettlement (WHO, 2007).

○ WHO ethical and safety recommendations for interviewing trafficked women. These guidelines include recommendations for conducting research with women and girls in the particularly sensitive area of trafficking and commercial sexual exploitation (Zimmerman and Watts, 2003).

Promote protection and participation

As has been highlighted throughout this book, research on violence against children with disabilities can be conducted directly with children, retrospectively with adults, indirectly through case review and analysis of administrative data or through interviews with caregivers, community members, professionals and key stakeholders. Any research on violence against children must constantly balance the rights to both participation and protection.

Children's involvement in research can be perceived in a variety of ways: children as objects, as subjects, as social actors and as active participants and co-researchers (Christensen and Prout, 2002). In the view of children as objects, children are regarded as dependent, incompetent and vulnerable beings, who are acted on by others and who lack the ability to consent or have their own voices in research. As a result, researchers carry out their research with adult-centred perspectives. Unfortunately, many studies in the area of child protection and disability adopt, often non-explicitly, the approach of children as objects of research.

Researchers who take the concept of children as subjects recognise a child's subjectivity. Children's involvement in research, however, is decided by researchers' judgements on children's cognitive abilities and social competencies. In this sense, researchers involve children in their research as informants and focus on assessing children's development and maturity (Yoon, 2016). These two concepts are not only the most traditional but are also adopted commonly among research related to children with disabilities.

Other perceptions of children and childhood, which are more participatory, are becoming increasingly common. One is the view of children as social actors with their own agency. In this way, children are positioned at the centre of research with their own experiences and understandings (Morrow, 2011). Thus, child-friendly research techniques and methods such as the examples provided in Chapters 3 and 4 are used to ensure children are engaged to speak about their own experiences and views. Best practice involves respecting the preferences of children with disabilities about how they want to participate in the research process.

Alongside the view of children as social actors, there is another concept of children as active participants. This describes research as a co-production by researchers and participants and further develops the perspective of children as co-researchers (see, for example, Bradbury-Jones, 2014). This emphasis on children's active involvement in research is aligned to the principle of children's right to participation enshrined in the United Nations Convention on the Rights of the Child (UNCRC), which has been ratified in almost every country. Particularly Article 12 states 'children have the right to say what they think should happen and have their opinions taken into account', while Article 13 recognises that children have the right to express their views and opinions, including in research, 'in any way they choose, including by talking, drawing or writing' (United Nations General Assembly, 1989).

This paradigm shifts from research 'on' children to research 'with' children with a growing interest in listening to children's experiences, and perspectives has increased over the past decade for research with children with disabilities (Gilligan, 2015). Therefore, in order to conduct ethical research, researchers need to consider how children participate as well as how they are protected during research.

In summary, the research must always balance respondents' right to participation while maintaining the highest level of child protection. While there has also been a gradual increase in research and attention in research ethics, it is still difficult to find research in which children with disabilities are involved more directly as active participants and where their participation rights are promoted actively alongside minimising risk and maximising protection.

Getting to know participants and assessing the risks

Information gathering and documentation must be done in a manner that presents the least risk to respondents, is methodologically sound and builds on current experience and good practice. Of the research case studies presented in this book, several good practice lessons can be shared:

- gather information in advance;
- work with implementing and disability-focused organisations; and
- work to limit potential risks.

In order to prepare the research best and to ensure both protection and participation, it is vital to gather information in advance about the context related to the research question, the potential participants and the methods that may be needed to ensure the research and consent processes are accessible to ensure active consent and participation (see Chapter 3 for examples).

The collection of information about violence against children with disabilities must be informed by a sound understanding of the culture and context within which the research is to take place. It must always be conducted in accordance with prescribed standards, principles and recommended good practice for working with survivors of violence (CP MERG, 2012). Involving local disability-focused and rights organisations, children's organisations or direct service providers, when it is safe to do so, is a good way to ensure that the proposed methodology is based on a sound understanding of the local context and is relevant and appropriate for the setting and respondents. This can also help to make sure that the required referral pathways are in place (see section on Accessible care and support referrals, below).

If local groups are to be approached and consulted in this way, it is considered best practice to learn something about the group(s) and their activities in advance of the research. It is also advisable to understand the limits to confidentiality that may exist in some smaller communities and to think carefully about employing interpreters or other members of the community in assisting with the research if it is likely to be perceived as a threat to the confidentiality of the participants (see section on Limits and challenges to privacy and confidentiality: Assessing risks). Also, in some settings characterised by complex political issues, there are likely to be some local groups whose involvement could result in harm to respondents and/or others involved in information collection activities (WHO, 2007). Gathering information in advance about settings, the context and local organisations will help to ensure the research is orientated to ensure safe and active participation.

Communication and coordination between organisations and researchers working on violence against children with disabilities should be promoted in order to avoid duplication of effort and to maximise the utility of existing data. It is unfair to ask children and communities to undergo repeated interviews and potentially repeated risks, for the convenience of multiple organisations and researchers (WHO, 2007). The purpose of the data to be collected on violence against children with disabilities should always be clearly defined and justified from the start of the study, and reviewed through independent ethical review processes, before any data collection takes place. Guidelines on other sensitive issues including violence against vulnerable groups highlight that it should also be demonstrated that the information to be gathered is not already available and/or does not exist in another form prior to commencing research (Zimmerman and Watts, 2003; WHO, 2007; CP MERG, 2012).

In summary, the benefits to respondents or communities of documenting violence against children with disabilities must be greater than the risks to respondents and communities.

Accessible care and support referrals

It may come to light during research that participants may be currently experiencing significant harm. This is especially the case when exploring issues and perceptions around violence. There is an ethical duty to ensure the safety of participants. Participants in research on violence – whether children or adults – may also wish to explore issues raised in the research with professionals such as counsellors or social workers. Often called 'referrals', it is important as a researcher to map out all the potential additional sources of information that may be needed and the professionals working in a range of areas, in case concerns about participant safety or well-being arise through the course of the research. Protection of children during the research process may involve making decisions about referrals, which researchers can experience as 'complex, fraught with ethical dilemmas and … a process of balancing risks and benefits of actions' (Gorin *et al.*, 2008, p. 284). Best practice highlights that research on violence must include information for all participants on a range of services including counselling for those who have experienced violence. However, dilemmas arise where referral services do not exist – for example, in rural areas in developing countries – or are not accessible to children with disabilities (Clacherty and Donald, 2007).

The case studies throughout this book highlight that the following steps are useful for ensuring appropriate referral pathways for research on violence against children with disabilities.

Be 'resource-ready' and identify available resources and support services in advance of data collection

Children with disabilities, their carers and family members as well as other adults may not have the possibility to access information that can benefit the health and safety of children with disabilities. An interviewer is responsible for providing information, as well as collecting it. An interview or data-collection situation is a good opportunity for a participant to obtain information about support services and programmes in the community (WHO, 2007). Information should be presented in a concise and clear way and in an accessible format for participants (see Chapter 4 for examples).

Make contact with and know the organisations and people on your referral list

It is important to ensure that all the referral information provided is accurate and up to date. This can include checking phone numbers, contact people and websites to make sure they are functioning and to provide information that will be useful. It is also important to test the accessibility of referral services (buildings, hotlines, etc.) for the specific types of access and support that the study's participants may need. This is where working with a key implementing partner such as child protection, disability-specific or other civil society organisations as well as welfare services is helpful (see examples from the case studies in Chapter 4).

Be prepared to 'fill the gaps' in the referral services

Several case studies mentioned the importance of dual training for referral providers. For example, an introduction and key overview on child protection may need to be provided to disability-specific organisations or training on disabilities to child protection organisations (Taylor *et al.*, 2014). Ideally, this should be done in collaboration with existing organisations and actors, but it is important not to make assumptions about the level of expertise in either child protection or disability on the part of referral organisations. Researchers should investigate this in advance and provide the additional information that these organisations may need to provide the best services to potential participants.

Develop referral pathways for different scenarios and identify a 'named person'

It is important not only to develop a list of referral resources in advance of data collection but also to think through potential disclosure scenarios and how the research team would handle these. The scenarios should include all of the populations included in the study (not just children) and cover a range of harmful situations that could come to light during the research, including both child and adult protection (for example, domestic abuse situations and suicide ideation).

Once these scenarios are developed, the research team can then plan the referral pathways for each scenario. Who will make a decision on when local authorities are called for significant harm cases? What referrals should be made for whom? This may involve identifying a 'named person' during the design stage of the study who can provide advice to the research team and be competent to make referral decisions. Often this may be a social worker or other professional who is familiar with the laws of the country in which the study is taking place as well as with the issue of child protection and disability. This person can act as a sounding board for difficult referral decisions. Examples from previous studies include utilising social welfare or local authority child protection officers (Taylor *et al.*, 2014) or organisations such as UNICEF who work on child protection with government and service providers. It is important to identify the various limits to confidentiality that the research team has agreed in their referral pathways, as well as anyone who will be acting as a 'named person' in the participant information sheet and consent forms.

Figure 5.2: What if referral services for children with disabilities who have experienced violence do not exist or are not functioning?

Asking questions about violence may result in some interviewees disclosing previous violence experiences. For some, this may be the first time they have told anyone about the incident, and they may want and need emotional support and help with any security and safety concerns. For others, the questions and discussion may bring forth emotional responses that require follow up and psychosocial assistance or healthcare beyond the scope of the interviewer's work. For these reasons, it is an ethical imperative that when conducting data collection activities appropriate follow-up referral information is provided.

However, throughout this book we have highlighted the barriers that exist in child protection and other services for responding to cases of violence against children with disabilities. How ethical is it then to undertake research on violence against children with disabilities if we know that specialist services are non-existent, care is substandard or the very services that are supposed to protect children are the ones perpetrating violence against children (such as police forces in some countries)? In order to make evidence-based recommendations for services, understanding the extent and nature of violence in the lives of children with disabilities is essential.

Ethical research requires that at least basic care and support services to which survivors (children or adult) may be referred must be available (WHO, 2007). Almost all countries have child protection systems – whether formalised through the state or through community-based child protection mechanisms. These systems are often supported by a range of international organisations and UN agencies, such as United Nations Children's Fund (UNICEF), that may also provide at least some of the services that a formal child protection system would provide.

In many countries, psychosocial support or counselling services for victims of violence will not be available or will be available only in urban centres. In order to overcome this challenge, some researchers employ their own social workers or certified counsellors to provide psychosocial support to participants if they want to talk to someone. Other strategies may include up skilling or training local community health workers in basic counselling techniques, or the commitment of government or private counselling services to support researchers and the participants (García-Moreno and Watts, 2004). These approaches, while overcoming ethical challenges for a specific study, do not provide longer-term solutions to inadequate care and protection of children in the country. Therefore, it is important if this method is employed to ensure that data that is collected is also utilised to help strengthen child protection systems and responses, as well as prevention approaches for children with disabilities (see section on Using the data and providing feedback to participants and communities).

In relatively isolated locations, or in the early stages of a humanitarian crisis (i.e. before relief efforts are fully operational), it is quite likely that no violence referral services whatsoever will be available. Under such circumstances, anyone gathering information about violence against children must follow international humanitarian minimum standards such as those developed for child protection in humanitarian contexts (CPWG, 2012).

In summary, researchers should plan in advance for referrals and ensure that basic follow-up care can be provided for all study participants.

Selecting and preparing interpreters, researchers and co-workers on child protection and disabilities

The case studies and research presented in this book highlight how important it is for anyone involved in the research team to have an understanding of both child protection and disability when undertaking research on violence against children with disabilities. Bespoke training for all those involved in the study, from research assistants to interpreters to drivers, should be made available. The findings highlighted through this book have identified twelve key areas for which training should be provided when researching in the area of violence against children with disabilities. The recommendations are:

- background to the areas of child protection and disability that are relevant to the study;
- background on purpose of study and on data collection and design and how the data will be used and presented back to the community;
- a review of the data-collection tools including how to ensure these tools and activities are accessible to participants. This may involve using role-playing activities to practise using the tools for the variety of scenarios and participants who may be included in the study;
- the study safeguarding and referral pathways including discussion of scenarios and what protocol the different members of the research team should follow in alerting the principal investigator and/or 'the named person' to child protection concerns;
- the procedures for and importance of maintaining confidentiality;
- the importance of securing and maintaining privacy during the interview;
- referral services and 'checking-in' to ensure ongoing consent and also the welfare of participants throughout the study;
- avoidance of personal and social harm to participants and researchers;
- the impact of 'vicarious' trauma for interviewers, self-care, team debriefings, referral services and procedures for the research team about engaging with the difficult topic of violence against children with disabilities;
- logistics of the data collection and standard operating procedures (SoPs);
- how to maintain and assess quality assurance and quality control of data;
- data protection procedures in the design, conduct, analysis and dissemination of findings.

Working with interpreters, or professionals who are used to mediating communication between people who do not use the same language, requires special attention when considering the ethical and methodological challenges of research on violence against children with disabilities. In most countries, interpreters are professionally trained and expected to adhere to a Code of Conduct or Code of Ethics. Codes for spoken and signed language interpreters incorporate the same tenets – maintaining impartiality and confidentiality, upholding a professional distance and interpreting faithfully and accurately (Mikkelson, 2000; Rodriguez and Guerrero, 2002). In early studies, interpreters were thought to be engaged only in passing information back and forth and were seen as being 'invisible' and not having impact on the message (Napier et al., 2010). However, research has shown that the very act of interpreting is to act as a participant in an interaction to co-construct meaning in language (Roy, 2000).

Sign language interpreters allow research to become accessible to participants who have additional support needs and require mediated conversation; some studies may choose to employ interpreters as part of the research team: for example, if they have non-deaf researchers who will be interacting with deaf participants. Interpreters should be given the research materials (questions, consent forms and other documents) in advance of the data collection in order to allow them time to prepare for interpreting. Researchers should also meet the interpreters and ask them if they have any questions on the study materials and talk to them about how best to organise the interview space. For studies that employ interpreters as part of the research team, it is essential those interpreters are part of the research training specified above and that they also understand the safeguarding and referral protocols for the study. Vicarious trauma of sign language interpreters is also a key issue to discuss and explore through the training.

For studies being undertaken in a specific geographic area, it might be good to ensure that interpreters do not know the research participants in order to help maintain privacy and confidentiality. Interpreters would be expected to follow the same privacy and confidentiality procedures as any other researcher in the study, and most interpreters will be familiar with the importance of confidentiality as a part of their professional standards.

In summary, comprehensive training covering the background of child protection and disability, the study protocol, safeguarding and referral pathways as well as data protection should be provided for all members of the research team including interpreters.

Accessible information and consent procedures

The role of informed consent is critical to ensuring study participants understand the purpose and content of the research, the procedures that will be followed and also their rights for participation.
The informed consent process is crucial and should be considered an
ongoing process throughout the life of the study and not a one-off event
(Graham *et al.,* 2013). Careful attention must be paid as to how information is given, considering issues of power and control in the setting
as well as the additional support needs of respondents (see Chapter 4
for a detailed discussion).

For child participants, consent procedures must be designed with
their specific needs, age and level of understanding in mind. Consent
policies and procedures relating to children should comply with existing local and national laws and policies. Some countries such as the
US will have federally mandated ethical review processes and procedures through IRBs – such boards are also often called Research Ethics
Boards or Committees depending on the country context. Care must
be taken to ensure that any study seeks the appropriate approvals to
undertake the research from ethical review boards at national, institutional and/or professional levels (e.g. for research with professionals,
additional ethical review approvals may be required, for example, with
teachers, social workers and health officials).

Information about the research activities should be provided to children and their parent or guardian in a manner that is appropriate to
their culture, education and level of understanding and communication. This is a key consideration to be taken into account when researching violence against children with disabilities and is where having a
research advisory committee comprising experts and key stakeholders is helpful to researchers to ensure quality of engagement. Consent
procedures, particularly how potential risks are described, will be different for adults and children. For children, it is important to ensure
that all materials and procedures are age-appropriate. In this regard,
dialogic consent, as explained in Chapter 4, may be particularly useful
for exploring the participant's understanding of the consent process. It
also allows for questions and dialogue about the study and the implications for participating. An excellent compendium of case studies
exists through the Ethical Research Involving Children website (www.

childethics.com, accessed 31 January 2017), which details different approaches in practice to key ethical and methodological issues in studies involving children.

It is critical during the informed consent process that researchers explain to all participants:

- the reason for the interview/survey/study;
- the subject matters to be discussed;
- the potential risk and benefits involved in participating including confidentiality procedures and any limits to confidentiality;
- the personal, and possibly upsetting, nature of any questions that may be asked (WHO, 2007).

It may also be beneficial for the interviewer to ask the participant to repeat back in her/his own way of communicating why the interview is being done, what she/he has agreed to, what the risks might be and what would happen if she/he refuses (see Figure 5.4; Zimmerman and Watts, 2003). In other words, the interviewer must carefully assess each aspect of the participant's understanding and explain or rephrase the information as many times as required (ibid.).

Parental consent and child assent

A parent or guardian for children under eighteen should provide informed consent for their child to participate in the study, unless local laws state otherwise (Graham *et al*, 2013). In addition, children who are of an age to be able to understand the nature of the information-gathering activity (i.e. are developmentally capable) must also give their consent to participate (see Chapter 3 for a more detailed discussion on 'capacity' to consent). In many countries, if an activity is deemed by experts in child rights/protection to have minimal risks (for example, an interview in a fairly stable setting with appropriate safeguards to protect participant's safety and confidentiality), parental consent may not be required for older adolescents. The process of determining acceptable and appropriate ages when adolescents may be able to give consent without parental involvement requires understanding of the applicable laws, culture and context as well as careful evaluation of safety and other issues in the setting (WHO, 2007). Figure 5.3 highlights the guidelines for obtaining parental consent and child assent, provided by the NSPCC, one of the leading non-governmental organisations for child protection in the UK. The NSPCC is one of the only national child protection organisations globally that the authors are aware of that has an ethical review board for research, which ensures that all research undertaken and commissioned by the organisation adheres to the highest standards of ethical and methodological rigour. Figure 5.3 highlights the key considerations to be put in place to explore both the intersection between age and developmental capacity (for example, for participants with learning disabilities) and the recommendations for parental consent and child assent.

If there are mandatory reporting requirements in the setting on child abuse, this information must be disclosed to the adults (parents, professionals, etc.) and child involved in the study during the consent process. Similarly, it is recommended that all studies develop a child protection and referral pathway, regardless of whether there are mandatory child abuse reporting laws or not, and also disclose this to adults and children through the consent procedures.

Limits and challenges to privacy and confidentiality: Assessing risks

Preserving the confidentiality of personal information is one of the fundamental principles governing the collection of data about individuals (WHO, 2007). Any personal information that an individual discloses in an information collection exercise should be considered to be confidential. This means that there is an implicit understanding that the disclosed information will not be shared with others, unless the person concerned gives explicit and informed consent to do so – thus highlighting the need to be explicit in study information and consent procedures about any limits to confidentiality for child protection purposes.

The requirement to maintain confidentiality governs not only how the data is collected (e.g. through conducting interviews in private spaces) but also how the data is stored (e.g. without names and other identifiers) and how the data is shared. The study protocol, which should be developed before the research starts, should explicitly highlight the procedures for maintaining confidentiality. Some key aspects to consider include the following.

Figure 5.3: Framework for Consent with Child and Young People (written by Nick Drey, Caroline Bryson, Steven Webster and Matt Barnard from the NSPCC; adapted and reprinted with approval from the NSPCC).

Age	Learning difficulty (LD)?	Capacity to give informed consent*? (Lack of capacity may be due to age, cognition or other factor)	Consent process (A child or young person's refusal of assent or consent should always overrule parent or guardian's consent to take part in research)
Under 8	With or without LD	Capacity to consent is unlikely	Parental consent, plus child's assent**
8–12	With or without LD	Capacity	Parental consent, plus child's consent
		No capacity	Parental consent, plus child's assent**
13–15	No LD	Assume all in this age group without LD have capacity to consent, unless otherwise indicated	Parental consent, and young person's consent
	LD	Capacity	Parental consent, plus young person's consent
	LD	No capacity	Parental consent, plus young person's assent**
16 or 17	No LD	Assume all in this age group without LD have capacity to consent, unless otherwise indicated	Young person's consent (We would encourage parental consent as well, if appropriate, for young people age 16–17)
	LD	Capacity	Parental consent, plus young person's consent
	LD	No capacity	Parental consent, plus young person's consent
18+	No LD	Capacity	Adult's consent
	LD	Capacity	Adult's consent
	LD	No capacity	This may require additional approval and ethical review under the remit of adult services in the particular country

* *Informed consent* is the voluntary agreement of an individual who has the legal capacity to give consent and who exercises free power of choice without undue inducement or any other form of constraint or coercion to participate in research. The individual must have sufficient knowledge and understanding of the nature of the proposed research, the anticipated risks and potential benefits, and the requirements of the research to be able to make an informed decision (Levine, 1988).

** *Assent* is defined as the child or young person's permission or affirmative agreement to participate in research (Broome and Richards, 1998). The seeking of assent may vary from situation to situation. It may approximate the consent process in an older adolescent child; with a younger child or a child or young person with significant learning difficulties assent may be established through ensuring that the child or young person is not troubled or disturbed by the research.

Choosing participants

Specific disabilities may make someone identifiable, so it is important to choose a large enough geographic area and/or sample size to ensure confidentiality for the participants in the study.

Issues related to privacy

Both children and adults with disabilities may require additional support from parents/carers, interpreters or other professionals to participate in research. This in addition to violence being a sensitive topic presents specific challenges for maintaining the privacy of the participants. For example, when planning to conduct interviews with children with disabilities, the dynamics of whether or not to have a parent present are an important consideration. In some cases, parents can provide support with their child's preferred communication method and the child may choose to have their parent present as they are a trusted adult who knows them well. However, children with disabilities should still have the same opportunities to express a preference about whether they would like their parent (or any other adult) present during a research interview (see Figure 5.4).

Limits to confidentiality

The referral pathways for potential scenarios for all participants and where possible limits to confidentiality exist for child protection purposes.

Standard operating procedures for breaches to confidentiality

Steps should be taken in the event of a breach of confidentiality and also its consequences. Penalties for breaches of confidentiality should be enforced.

Developing participant ID numbers

The names of participants should not be used on forms or in documents or other types of written or electronic materials generated as part of the study. Instead, participants should be given ID numbers, and the document linking the participant name with the ID number should be stored separately from the data. If follow-up is required for referrals or safeguarding, these ID numbers can be used in research documents.

Training on confidentiality

Training should be provided for all members of the research team on the need for and procedures to maintain confidentiality. As part of this training, potential role-play or case-study scenarios could be explored to enhance the training (see, for example, Figure 5.4, which would be an excellent training case study for discussion). Discussion on the practical applications of confidentiality principles in the setting in which they will be working should also be explored: for example, if visiting a small village for data collection, highlighting the steps researchers should follow to maintain confidentiality.

Considerations on employing local members of the research team

Thought should be given to the confidentiality issues in settings where the researchers and other team members are drawn from the community or are living within the community that is part of the planned investigation (WHO, 2007). Under these circumstances, training programmes should explore the challenges local staff may face in maintaining confidentiality on a day-to-day basis and provide strategies for addressing these issues (WHO, 2007). Careful consideration should be given as to whether interviewers, translators, transcribers, interpreters or other team members should work within their own communities, especially when researching the area of violence against children with disabilities.

Confidentiality agreements

Where required and useful, team members including transcribers and translators and advisory committee members can sign confidentiality agreements. These should highlight the expectations required of the person in terms of maintaining confidentiality including by destroying documents after review, not sharing information and specifying safe storage of documents. Contents of individual interviews should be discussed only with others who are bound by the same duty of confidentiality, and then only when necessary. Interview contents should never be discussed in public, particularly where they can be overheard: for example, in the presence of taxi drivers (Zimmerman and Watts, 2003).

Storage of data

All completed forms, records, photographs, audiotapes, videotapes, flip-chart papers, etc. should be stored and confidentially labelled as soon as possible after use in a secure location, ideally in locked cabinets. Only a limited number of people should have access to these secured storage facilities. As camp or field settings are rarely secure, additional measures may be needed to ensure the personal safety of those staff with access to the data storage areas (Zimmerman and Watts, 2003). Suitable arrangements must also be made if at any time materials have to be moved to other locations. Indexes for matching code numbers with identifying information/names should always be stored separately and securely.

Destroying the data

Audio and video recordings of interviews should be destroyed once a transcript of the interview has been created or within the timeframe specified by the governing IRB. If audiotape or videotape is made for purposes other than simply recording an interview, the person responsible must not only justify why it needs to be made but also make provision for preserving the confidentiality of those featured in the recording (WHO, 2007).

Figure 5.4: Case study – Issues related to privacy with parents and carers.

This case study is drawn from a research study by Berni Kelly that examined the provision of family support services for children with intellectual disabilities (e.g. learning disabilities) in Northern Ireland. A key objective of the research was to ascertain the views of children and consult with them about their experiences of family support services.

The ethical challenge

The study involved interviews with children with intellectual disability over the course of three visits in the family home. Before visiting children, the researcher discussed the research process with parents and explained that some children may wish their parent to be present and others may not. The researcher explained that the child would make a decision on this matter, but would also be free to change their mind. On first visits, the researcher consulted each child about their preference of being interviewed on their own or having their parent present. In one case a child indicated a preference to meet the researcher on their own.

The researcher informed the parent of their child's preference and agreed with the parent that they would see their child alone on the next visit. On the second visit, after welcoming the researcher into the family home, the parent continued to stay in the same room with the child and researcher. The researcher was unsure if the parent had forgotten their earlier discussion about meeting their child on their own or if they still assumed they should remain present. The researcher had to decide how best to address this issue without causing distress for either the child or parent. She was also mindful that her response to this ethical dilemma would send a message to the child about whether the researcher respected and prioritised their views and preferences, which could impact on the child's participation in the interview.

The researcher could proceed with the interview and ignore the issue of parental presence unless the child raised it as a problem. This approach would avoid confrontation and ensure the parent did not feel excluded. However, this method would fail to prioritise the child's preference and could impact on their interview responses as the adult present would be in control of the research process. Instead, the researcher could speak with the parent on their own to explain the research process again and offer them an opportunity to discuss any concerns. However, this may lead the child to believe that the adults are privately discussing their involvement in the research and reaching a decision without including them. An alternative choice would be to address the issue with the child and parent both present. This option may lead the child to feel that they have upset their parent by excluding them and to feel pressured to change their mind. However, this approach would ensure that the issue is addressed in a transparent way with both the child and the parent.

Choices made

The researcher decided on the last option, with both the child and the parent present. She took great care to approach the subject in a sensitive and supportive manner. Explaining that the child's views were the main priority for the researcher and reminding the child and parent about the child's expressed preference on the previous visit was a good starting point. The parent explained that they had become accustomed to remaining present during visits from professionals as it was usually assumed that they would provide information on behalf of their child, especially when there were concerns that their child may not be able to answer some questions. The researcher explained the purpose of the research again and emphasised that she was primarily interested in their child's views and it was fine if their child was not able to answer all of the questions or did not wish to answer some questions. The child also advised their parent that they felt comfortable being on their own with the researcher as a range of communication tools were provided to support their participation, including drawing, sentence completion, computer-assisted techniques and sign cards. Following this discussion, the parent was happy to leave the room and for their child to meet the researcher on their own for the next two visits.

Case study discussion questions

○ What could the researcher have done if the child or parent became upset during the discussion about the child being interviewed alone?

○ If the parent insisted on being present, what could the researcher do? Would it be appropriate to conduct the child's interview with the parent present, knowing that it was not the child's preferred approach?

○ In cases where children prefer their parent to be present, what techniques could the researcher use to ensure the views of the child are prioritised?

○ What are the risks for the researcher when meeting children on their own?

Case study printed with permission from the author, Dr Berni Kelly, Senior Lecturer at Queen's University Belfast. Permission was also received from the Centre for Children and Young People, Southern Cross University, which manages the compendium of case studies for the Ethical Research Involving Children website, through which this case study was first published. Further case studies can be found at www.childethics.com (accessed 31 January 2017).

Going at the child's pace and avoiding re-traumatising the child

When involving children with disabilities in research, it is important to go at their pace and to design data-collection activities according to their development stage and with additional support needs in mind. In order to accomplish this, two recent studies in Scotland on child protection and disability have utilised a two-meeting approach called 'guided conversations' (Stalker *et al.*, 2010; Taylor *et al.*, 2015a). The first meeting was held with a child as an introductory session with the objective of checking that the child understood what the project was about and had an opportunity to ask any questions. This also allowed researchers to establish the communication methods supplemented by additional communication information collected prior to the first meeting and to decide what materials should be used at the data-collection session (e.g. the second meeting) (Stalker *et al.*, 2010). The second meeting was designed to check consent again for participation in the study and to conduct the interview. In a recently published report, it was documented that the young people preferred to continue with data collection at the first meeting and did not want or need a second meeting (Taylor *et al.*, 2015a).

Icebreakers have been identified by several case studies within this book as being important for establishing rapport and trust with participants before asking questions or commencing data collection. Various icebreaker activities exist and can include giving the child an opportunity to undertake a creative activity such as drawing a picture along the lines of 'something that is important to me' (Stalker *et al.*, 2010) or another activity aimed at getting to know the other participants.

Use of direct interviewing

Throughout the case studies in this book, challenges have been raised about the direct involvement of children with disabilities in interviewing. As with all violence-related research, special attention should be paid to activities that involve the interviewing of survivors or those who may have experienced any form of violence during childhood. Promising practices highlight that personal interviews should be used only to obtain information after all other options have been considered. While balancing the rights to participation, researchers should consider the following before engaging in the methodological approach of direct interviewing:

- that the desired data cannot be collected without gathering information in this way;
- that the potential respondents and the larger community want to participate;
- that the information is needed and is not otherwise already available;
- that information cannot be obtained in a less invasive manner (e.g. by using other methods or approaches with lower risk);
- that participants can fully understand and engage in the research;
- that the welfare of respondents and communities can be properly protected throughout the research study period and beyond.

Appropriately handling disclosures during interviews

It is important to recognise that some participants will experience some level of stress or discomfort when discussing certain issues related to violence. Part of the training for team members involved in this area of research is to be comfortable with emotions and also to recognise when to stop an interview. For many respondents, it can also be therapeutic to discuss these issues and to be listened to (Campbell, 2002). Participants should always be offered referral and support service information.

A respondent may disclose experiencing violence in the past or currently during the course of the data collection. It is important to note that this may be the first time the respondent is telling anyone about the violence he or she has experienced (Campbell, 2002). Extensive research on responding to disclosures by survivors of violence highlights that the response to disclosures can determine whether a survivor ever tells anyone ever again about the violence or if they decide to seek support services (McElvaney *et al.*, 2014; Alaggia, 2010; Aherns, 2006). Thus, an interviewer's response to disclosures is incredibly important for the welfare of participants (see Figure 5.5).

Figure 5.5: Handling disclosures of past violence experiences during data collection.

How disclosures are handled is incredibly important as to whether someone ever tells anyone again about the violence they have experienced. This book has highlighted the barriers that exist for people with disabilities who have experienced violence during childhood, as also highlighted in Chapter 2. It is important that these disclosures are appropriately and sensitively handled during the research process as such, and that researchers have child protection training that covers handling disclosures. The following steps can be explored if a participant discloses having ever experienced violence during an interview or through participation in any data collection activity:

○ *Listen:* Suspend the research for the time being and actively listen to the participant.

○ *Acknowledge:* Identify what the person is saying in a sensitive manner (do not ignore what they just said!). The interviewer could say something like: 'Thank you for sharing this with me, I know it takes tremendous courage to share your own personal experience.'

○ *Provide referral:* At the end of the interview, give the participant the prepared referral information or follow safeguarding procedures if it comes to light that a child or young person is currently at risk of significant harm

○ *Decide whether to continue or end the interview/survey:* Use best judgement about whether to continue with the survey. It is important to recognise that asking a respondent (adult or child) to share information on a sensitive subject and then interrupting that story or expressions of emotion or ending the interview/data collection before they have had a chance to complete their thoughts can be upsetting (WHO, 2007). However, if a respondent becomes very distressed or overwhelmed (e.g., displaying some of the following symptoms: trembling or shaking, crying uncontrollably), it is best to inquire whether the respondent prefers to carry on, to change the subject or to terminate the interview or survey (WHO, 2007).

○ *Thank the respondent:* Thank the respondent again for sharing their experience and inform them of any plans for sharing the findings of the study with the community.

In summary, careful consideration should be given to designing research and whether direct interviewing is the most appropriate approach to collecting data on violence against children with disabilities. Data collectors should also be trained on how appropriately to handle disclosures of either current or past experiences of violence that respondents may recount.

Quality assurance mechanisms

Quality assurance during research is the systematic process of checking to see that all steps of the research being developed are meeting the specific ethical, quality and safety recommendations. The following mechanisms are examples of processes that can enhance quality assurance for researching violence against children with disabilities:

• Utilise a research advisory group composed of key academics, programme staff and policymakers in the area of child protection and disability as well as people with disabilities who can act as a sounding board and monitoring body for ethical issues throughout the research. This group should have the opportunity to review and comment on all study-related materials including consent forms and procedures, study instruments and final reports and dissemination materials.

• Hold regular research team meetings that can serve as a quality assurance channel in that, at these meetings, progress against set milestones and agreed ethical, quality and safety procedures can be regularly reviewed. These meetings can also serve as opportunities for identifying, discussing and debriefing on matters arising related to ethical issues.

• Training should be held for all those involved in data collection to ensure consistency in approach and quality across the study, including sensitivity to participants' needs.

• By engaging with these and other recommendations for quality assurance, the ethical, quality and safety issues can be regularly assessed throughout the research cycle and corrective action taken at the earliest possible opportunity if issues arise.

Vicarious trauma in the research team

Researchers working in the area of research on violence against children with disabilities are exposed to disturbing stories of violence, humiliation and abuse throughout the process of collecting, analysing and reporting on their data (Coles *et al.*, 2010). This research can lead to secondary traumatic stress or what is often called 'vicarious trauma'. Vicarious trauma can be defined as the transformation of the researcher's inner experience as a result of empathetic and/or repeated engagement with trauma material such as that often gathered through violence against children studies (Pearlman and Saakvitne, 1995; Coles *et al.*, 2010).

In a study of the impact of vicarious trauma on sexual violence researchers, it was found that many felt ill prepared for the emotional impact of the research they were undertaking (Coles *et al.*, 2010). The most common emotional responses described were anger, guilt, fear, sadness, crying and feeling depressed as well as experiencing nightmares, being irritable, having intrusive thoughts and difficulty concentrating. Researchers also described the impact of the exploring these issues on their worldview and a shift in deeming the world as an unsafe and dangerous place, because of their painful awareness of the extent of harm and suffering inflicted by the perpetrators of violence (Coles *et al.*, 2010).

Many strategies can be employed by researchers themselves to counteract the impact of the emotional stress of exposure to data on violence against children. 'Self-care' strategies can include spending time with friends and family and engaging in hobbies and activities that bring pleasure. It is important to note that anyone exposed to the material – including translators, transcribers and interpreters – can experience vicarious trauma.

Research managers and study investigators have an important role to play to ensure the safety and well-being of their team (Campbell, 2002). This includes time management and monitoring exposure of team members to traumatic material in all stage of the research from fieldwork to data entry to analysis and report writing. Ensuring the study findings are utilised to 'make a difference' was also cited as a key strategy to reduce vicarious trauma (Coles *et al.*, 2010). Another key strategy is holding regular 'debrief' meetings of the team, an open space to speak about the impact of doing the studies (Campbell, 2002).

In addition to training of team members in vicarious trauma and researcher safety, those undertaking this difficult work must also reflect on their capacity to engage with this material (Coles *et al.*, 2010). Best practice highlights that the opting out by researchers who feel 'at risk' should be seen as appropriate practice and be advised and supported by supervisors, managers and their organisations (Coles *et al.*, 2010; Campbell, 2002). Organisations supporting research on violence against children with disabilities have a duty of care and should respond to trauma among their team members. Finally, protocols should also include a dedicated section on safety that addresses the study procedures for working with sensitive material and supporting team members throughout the study (Dickson-Swift *et al.*, 2005).

In summary, all researchers and team members exposed to the stories and data on violence against children with disabilities may experience vicarious trauma. Protocols, training and self-care strategies should be employed to ensure the safety and well-being of the team.

Using the data and providing feedback to participants and communities

The experiences related to violence against children with disabilities should be gathered for a purpose. The enormous personal, social and health-related costs of violence against children, and the increased risk of this violence against children with disabilities, place a moral obligation on the researcher to make certain that the information collected is used to benefit respondents and also brought to the attention of policymakers and advocates (UNICEF, 2012; CP MERG, 2012).

Best practice, as evidenced through many of the case studies presented throughout this book, highlights that results of research findings should be presented in accessible ways to communities that participated in the study. This could include engaging young people through child-friendly methods and approaches to engage with the findings as well as involving policymakers and key stakeholders in order to validate and reflect on the findings before they are published to a wider audience.

Research should also be conducted in such a way as to maximise benefit to survivors of violence, participants and the community. For example, results should be made available in safe and ethical ways to community programmes that help prevent and respond to violence against children or those who work with children with disabilities in order to support the case for new or improved interventions. In addition, researchers must be certain that any information released publicly through reports, news releases and public statements are not misinterpreted and do not fuel prejudices or stereotypes against people with disabilities.

Conclusion

The key areas of good practice and subsequent recommendations detailed in this chapter reflect current knowledge and lessons learnt about the ethical and safety considerations to be addressed when undertaking research related to violence against children with disabilities. By prioritising the safety of children and communities, researchers can make significant contributions to the public recognition of the serious issue of violence against children with disabilities in order to ensure that all children have access to the best care and to provide evidence-based information to help prevent violence before it ever starts.

CHAPTER 6

Conclusion

Having accurate data on violence in the lives of children with disabilities is crucial. Throughout this book, we have highlighted the methodological and ethical challenges in designing, conducting, analysing and disseminating research on violence against children with disabilities.

The limits of our knowledge

In reviewing the prior research on violence in the lives of children with disabilities, most sources agree that children with disabilities are at higher risk for victimisation and face more severe victimisation.

While it is apparent that children with disabilities are at higher risk, the extent of that risk remains unclear because of challenges associated with collecting data on victimisation in general and specifically among children with disabilities. A review of the data sources available indicated a need for both nationally representative data with an oversample of children with disabilities that will allow for a type-specific analysis as well as qualitative data to understand the nature of violence and barriers to services and appropriate responses. In addition, future research needs to address directly the time dimension of the complex relationship between disability and victimisation, to determine which is the antecedent and which is the outcome.

Our limited understanding about the extent of the relationship between disability and victimisation also reflects a system that is ill-equipped to provide services and support to children with disabilities. The lack of disability-specific data available in child protective service reports reflects a problem for researchers in terms of data but more importantly highlights a systemic issue that disability is not being addressed/acknowledged within the system. If case workers are not mentioning disability in reports, this likely means that the caseworkers are also lacking resources and training on disability-specific issues.

A key topic throughout the interviews was the ethically difficult decision and concerns around direct interviews. This has been discussed for research with children in general, and extensively so when considering research with children on a sensitive topic such as exposure to violence (Knight *et al.*, 2000; Morris *et al.*, 2012). It became clear from studies in this field that the complexity of ethical considerations increases significantly when children have disabilities, particularly when it is unknown how an individual understands and processes potentially distressing information. In the case studies, this concern was handled methodologically in many different ways: by reducing or simplifying assessment; by retrieving information from case file reviews; by focusing direct questioning on court proceedings or perceived support, rather than on the offence itself; or by retrieving information from proxies or the community.

The ethical concern around the potential harms of research on the participating individuals was also reflected in carers' instincts to protect individuals with disabilities and not provide permission for them to be interviewed or surveyed directly.

Some of the case studies revealed that for ethical reasons some individuals with the most 'severe' disabilities who might be at highest risk had to be excluded from the research as it was impossible to ascertain that the individual understood the scope of research.

Overall, it was felt that it was important to have an ongoing dialogue with the IRB whenever possible, to discuss concerns, propose how to solve them, and to work on course correction when unexpected events took place in the field. This was particularly true when working in logistically challenging low-resource settings.

Practical concerns and challenges faced by researchers in the field

The methodological and ethical concerns were raised in Chapter 2, and recommendations for future work were extended upon through an examination of the case studies in Chapter 4. In attempting to gather information on the experience, challenges and lessons learnt when actually collecting data on victimisation in the lives of children with disabilities, we recognised that there was very little information available.

One of the key findings of these case studies, which was mirrored in several other studies, was the recommendation to include research expertise from both fields – disability and violence – so that challenges can be identified and solved jointly. In addition, in many cases it was reported to be beneficial to have the implementing organisation closely involved to help facilitate and train staff on how to interact with study participants, and specifically plan in time to break the ice. Furthermore, the importance of speaking the same language was mentioned several times, not only in relation to the actual spoken language but also when referring to using accessible not overly academic language that everyone understands.

Overall, the evidence suggests the importance of starting to compile systematic good practices as well as decisions that need to be taken and preparations required for future research, so that we can build momentum and increase the evidence base on this complex but important topic. Many of the lessons learnt from challenges faced by researchers, such as those related to informed consent, can also be extended to those working in the child welfare system.

Protecting children

Research on violence in the lives of children with disabilities is necessary and vital to understand the extent of the problem and to formulate solutions. As researchers we also need to protect children in research and also allow for their full participation.

Several examples were provided where the methodology was amended to allow children with disabilities to take part in the research. Adjustments naturally varied for the type of disability, each with different challenges that needed to be considered carefully. Some examples included: variation in the number of items used to assess violence that might affect prevalence rates (Thompson *et al.*, 2012); making sure that the item's purpose or an explanation remains the same even if simplified; and ensuring participant safety and confidentiality when choosing interpreters.

To have a strong referral system in place was determined to be essential and yet was challenging for many reasons, mostly related to accessibility. If research is conducted in a low-resource setting where no referral system exists, an organisation specialised in child protection might need to be tasked to take on this role for the duration of the research.

Recommendations for future areas of research

A number of key areas that need further research were also identified. Probably most pressingly, researchers need a better understanding of the consequences of participating in violence-related research, especially among children with disabilities. While we know little about the effects of responding to questions about victimisation in general, minimal research has been conducted involving children with disabilities. A better understanding of the risk associated with participating in research will enable us to weigh better the risks and benefits of research on violence against children, and to balance the principles of participation and protection.

To this end, there is also a need to develop indicators around capacity to consent to research. A more evidence-based model to determining capacity would alleviate some of the ethical issues researchers face when making these judgements, and would also be an important move towards ensuring certain children are not excluded from research.

More work is required on providing robust and disaggregated data that captures the experiences and nature of violence against children with disabilities across the lifespan. There is also a need for more research on the intersections between disability and gender and on how boys and girls with disabilities experience and respond to violence. Intersectionality research that addresses other dimensions such as race/ethnicity and socio-economic status would also be important to understand how these affect the relationship between violence and disability.

In addition, several discussions and considerations were noted around how to measure disability – specifically the lack of a universal definition of disability and the wide variation between measurements used. While most victimisation research among children with disabilities has used tools consistent with the medical model of disability, it is crucial that measurements take into account the intersections between an individual and the social and environmental factors that can create disabling barriers. This book has presented examples of how the social model of disability has been applied in child protection research, but it is important that these efforts be expanded.

Issues around categorising disability also arose, specifically whether to include learning disabilities, memory problems, concentration difficulties and emotional and behavioural problems. This in turn may have an impact on how disability is assessed, as some of these might not be detected in self-report, but may require additional sources of information such as from psychometric testing. Other topics related to measuring disability came up in relation to time-consistency of disability and the finding that some disabilities might change over time (they might arise as a result of an accident; some might be treatable or be detected only as the child grows older). The value of multi-informant assessment of disability was also demonstrated, as a higher correlation of disability between multiple informants may indicate an increased risk of exposure to violence. In addition, there was indication that impact of exposure to violence on a child with a disability might be related to the age of the child and how the child is able to process information. There was a perceived need to understand how evolving capacity and resiliency influence the impact of violence on the lives of children with disabilities.

Furthermore, the topic of social perception and/or myths arose. For some of the studies, this was an explicit part of the exploration. In others, it was clear that social perception shaped both fields – disability and violence against children – and some specifically related to the combined fields of violence against children with disabilities. Future efforts should increase our understanding of how these myths influence the process and the outcome of research, as well as how children with disabilities are treated within the child protection system (Reiman, 2014).

While research is emerging in the area of measuring the magnitude and scope of violence against children with disabilities as well as the effectiveness of existing programmes, more research is needed in order to ensure that no child is left behind in achieving the SDG to 'End abuse, exploitation, trafficking and all forms of violence against children' (United Nations General Assembly, 2015).

APPENDIX

Case studies

Please note: The authors obtained permission to print the information from these case studies from the researchers they interviewed. The conclusions of the researchers interviewed do not necessarily reflect the opinions of all principal investigators, research partners, publishers or funders.

Figure A.1: Chapter 4 case study details

Geographic region	Principal investigators	Interviewees	Description of research
United Kingdom	Anita Franklin, Phil Raws and Emilie Smeaton	Anita Franklin (31 March 2016)	This UK-wide study sought to understand the service-provision needs of young people with learning disabilities who have experienced or were at risk of child sexual exploitation (CSE) (Franklin et al., 2015). The research was conducted in partnership with Barnardo's and The Children's Society, two leading children's charities that runs most of the CSE services in the UK, as well as the British Institute of Learning Disabilities. Using mixed methods, the researchers sent surveys to local health authorities and relevant service providers across England, Scotland, Wales and Northern Ireland and conducted interviews with practitioners, and with young people identified to be at risk of or who had experienced CSE. Advisory groups – one professional reference group of practitioners and academics and the other comprising five young people with learning disabilities who had experienced CSE – were consulted on aspects of the study throughout
United States	Desmond Runyan, Howard Dubowitz, Mary Wood Schneider, Patrick Curtis, Jonathan Kotch, Alan Litrownik, Diana English, Wanda Hunter, Maureen Black, Raymond Starr, Jr, John Landsverk and David Marshall	Desmond Runyan (8 April 2016)	The Longitudinal Studies of Child Abuse and Neglect (LONGSCAN) began in the US in 1990. LONGSCAN is a group of research studies coordinated by a centre in North Carolina with five other sites around the country, each of which conducted a separate project on child maltreatment among a cohort of high-risk children while using common methods and analyses. It followed 1,354 children and their families who were recognised to be at risk of maltreatment or who had been maltreated in early childhood in order to understand long-term health outcomes of abuse and neglect. After baseline data was collected, children and their families were interviewed at ages four, six, eight, twelve, fourteen, sixteen and eighteen. Data on child maltreatment was obtained through several sources: from child protective services; teachers, parents or caregivers; and the young person from age twelve. A number of measures were used to assess children's development (Battelle scales), emotional and behavioural functioning (e.g., Vineland Adaptive Behaviour Scales) and overall health status (Child Health and Development). These were administered to parents or caregivers and teachers, and from age twelve the child. At ages four and six, questions about specific impairments were asked of parents or caregivers using the Child Health Assessment. At age four, the parent or caregiver was asked 'yes' or 'no' questions about whether the child had any of the following eight conditions: emotional disorder; mental retardation; developmental delay; physical handicap; hearing problem; speech problem; vision problem; and chronic illness/disease. At age six, the caregiver was asked if the child had been diagnosed with the following: hearing problem; speech or talking problem; vision or seeing problem; chronic health condition; physical handicap; hyperactivity or attention problem; learning problem; emotional problem; or mental retardation

Hong Kong	Ko Ling Chan, Clifton R. Emery and Patrick Ip	Ko Ling Chan (14 February 2016 and 7 March 2016)	A large survey of school-aged children in Hong Kong (n = 5,841, aged 9–18 years) aimed to provide reliable estimates of direct and indirect experiences of violence among children with disabilities, namely exposure to maltreatment, parental intimate partner violence and in-law conflict (Chan et al., 2014). The prevalence of disability among children was about 6% (n = 373), a rate comparable to the proportion of children with a disability found in the population. About 53.2% were boys. As a follow-up to this research, an additional study has been conducted, integrating lessons learnt (at the time of this chapter, data collection was just completed with an n of approximately 3,900 children). The study oversampled children with disability in order to increase the strength of the conclusions to include around 800 children with special needs (Chan et al., 2014). However, no results are available as of yet.
Burundi, Kenya and Rwanda	Handicap International and University of New South Wales	Sofia Hedjam and Sarah Rizk (2 February 2016)	As part of Handicap International's pilot implementation of the Ubuntu Care Project in Burundi, Kenya and Rwanda, it partnered the University of New South Wales to evaluate the project in Burundi as part of the Children and Violence Evaluation Challenge Fund. The aim of the project is a reduction of sexual violence against children, especially those with disabilities, by addressing the problem on an individual, community and national level. It empowers children to become key actors in their own protection while supporting other stakeholders (especially families) to create a safe protective environment. The evaluation focuses on measuring the change in attitudes, perceptions and behaviours as a result of intervention, and the underlying theory of change within the programme. The evaluation uses a mixed-method approach and a quasi-experimental design
Uganda	Karen M. Devries, Nambusi Kyegombe, Maria Zuurmond, Jenny Parkes, Jennifer C. Child, Eddy J. Walakira and Dipak Naker	Dipak Naker, Nambusi Kyegombe and Hannah Kuper (29 February 2016)	Between 2012 and 2014, Raising Voices' 'Good School Toolkit', a school-based violence prevention programme in Uganda, underwent a rigorous research evaluation conducted by the London School of Hygiene and Tropical Medicine. A total of 3,706 children and young adolescents aged 11–14 were randomly sampled from 42 primary schools in the Luwero district. The baseline survey revealed that approximately 9% of boys and 8% of girls reported a disability. Levels of violence against both children with and without disabilities were extremely high. Girls with disabilities reported slightly more physical (99.1% verdsus 94.6%, p = 0.010) and almost twice as much sexual violence (23.6% versus 12.3%, p = 0.002) than girls without disabilities; for boys with and without disabilities, levels are not statistically different
Switzerland	Manuel Eisner and Denis Ribeau	Manuel Eisner (31 January 2016 and 31 March 2016); data provided by Denis Ribeau and Margi Averdijk	The Zurich Project on the Social Development of Children in Zurich (z-proso) is an ongoing combined longitudinal and intervention study, which has been conducted in Switzerland since 2004. The target population for the study consisted of all 2,520 children who entered the first grade of public primary school in the city of Zurich in 2004. A stratified sample of fifty-six schools was drawn, comprising a final target sample of 1,675 children. The study has since been through seven annual or biannual data collection time points at ages seven, eight, nine, eleven, thirteen, fifteen and seventeen, the most recent being in 2015. The study has a special focus on 'violence' and 'aggressive behaviour', but it also comprises repeat measures of ADHD symptoms, non-aggressive conduct problems, delinquency, internalising symptoms and prosocial behaviour. From age seven, behaviour problems were assessed by administering the Social Behavior Questionnaire (Tremblay et al., 1992) to parents, teachers and children; violent and non-violent delinquency were assessed with a delinquency self-report questionnaire from age ten onwards. Only children that were able to attend public schools were included in the study. Children taught in small classes because of special educational needs are included, but children with 'severe' disabilities were as a result of the nature of the sample excluded. Children that became disabled later in life, for example as a result of an injury, continued to be part of the sample and were followed. See maim text for detailed results

Results from the z-proso study: Multi-informant reports of disability status

Primary caregivers were asked about the child's disability at age seven (wave 1) by assessing whether the child at the time of the interview had any of the following health issues: a visual or hearing impairment; a severe chronic illness leading to regular hospitalisation; any other physical disability; an intellectual disability; a delayed physical development;

or a delayed intellectual development. Responses were given in a yes/no format, with a request to specify if the answer was yes. This case study presents previously unpublished data on child protection and disability from this important research. The prevalence of parent-assessed disabilities at age seven can be seen in Figure A.2.

Figure A.2: Prevalence of disabilities in the sample according to the parents of a child aged seven (n = 1,235).

	n (%)
Vision or hearing impairment	124 (10.0%)
Severe chronic illness that results in regular hospitalisation	30 (2.4%)
Other physical disability	29 (2.3%)
Intellectual disability	3 (0.2%)
Physical developmental delay	52 (4.2%)
Intellectual developmental delay	83 (6.7%)
Any	273 (22.1%)

Eight years later, at the age of fifteen years (wave six of the longitudinal study), a brief disability-assessment was administered to the children as part of a paper-and-pencil questionnaire. Respondents were asked to assess whether they had any six persistent health problems that made it difficult for them to do the activities that others of their age did. The disability domain was similar, but not identical to those included in the parent questionnaire, namely: a visual impairment (only if persisting after usual correction); a hearing impairment; a lower limb disability; an upper limb disability; learning, memory and concentration problems; and a communicative disability (see Figure A.3).

Figure A.3: Prevalence of disabilities in the sample according to the youths at T6 (n = 1,447).

	n (%)
Visual impairment	37 (2.6%)
Hearing impairment	7 (0.5%)
Lower limb disability	5 (0.3%)
Upper limb disability	10 (0.7%)
Cognitive disability	160 (11.1%)
Communicative disability	42 (2.9%)
Any	221 (15.4%)

The two measures correlate very poorly:

- T1–T6 physical disability   0.083 (p = 0.005)
- T1–T6 mental/cognitive disability   0.055 (p = 0.067)

- T1–T6 any disability   0.086 (p = 0 .004)

Correlation for most measures is near zero, and even for those measures that show a statistically significant correlation the correlation is low. To some extent, the small correlations may have been affected by some differences in the item wording. However, the questions asked of the mother when the child was aged seven and those used in the child-questionnaire at age fifteen were similar enough to expect substantially higher correlations.

To explore possible reasons for the low correlations further, the authors first dichotomised 'any' disability according to the mother report (age seven of the child) and self-report (age fifteen), and then created a four-fold variable that was coded as:

    0 = not disabled, both informants (n = 756)

    1 = disabled mother report, not disabled child report (n = 189)

    2 = not disabled mother report, disabled child report (n = 119)

    3 = disabled, both reports (n = 52)

A series of analysis of variance (ANOVA) was subsequently conducted to explore whether disability reported by the mother, and disability reported by the child were predictive of criterion outcomes at age fifteen. The focus was on measures of internalising symptoms (anxiety/depression) and measures of victimisation:

- Teacher-assessed internalising symptoms at age fifteen varied signifwicantly between groups $(F(3,975) = 11.58, p < 0.0001)$. Both informants contributed to variation in internalising symptoms. They were highest when both informants agreed (M = 1.12), second highest if the child only reported disability (M = 1.06), and lowest if both informants did not see a disability (M = 0.76). They were also elevated if only the mother reported a disability when the child was aged seven (M = 1.01).
- Self-reported bullying victimisation at age fifteen was also highest if both informants reported a disability.
- Measure of disability assessed by the mother of child age seven did not predict serious violent victimisation reported by the adolescent at age fifteen. In contrast, self-reported violent victimisation was predicted by concurrent self-reported disability.

REFERENCES

Aherns, C. E. (2006) 'Being silenced: The impact of negative social reactions on the disclosure of rape', *American Journal of Community Psychology*, Vol. 38, pp. 263–74; doi:10.1007/s10464–006–9069–9

Alaggia, R. (2010) 'An ecological analysis of child sexual abuse disclosure: Considerations for child and adolescent mental health', *Journal of the Canadian Academy of Child and Adolescent Psychiatry*, Vol. 19, No. 1

Alderson, P. (1995) *Listening to Children: Children, Ethics and Social Research*, London: Barnardos

Alderson, P. (2004) 'Ethics', in Fraser, S., Lewis, V., Ding, S., Kellett, M. and Robinson, C. (eds.) (2004) *Doing Research with Children and Young People*, London: Sage

Alderson, P. and Morrow, V. (2006) 'Multidisciplinary research ethics review: Is it feasible?', *International Journal of Social Research Methodology*, Vol. 9, No. 5; doi:10.1080/13645570500435207

Allnock, D. and Miller, P. (2013) 'No one noticed, no one heard: A study of disclosures of childhood abuse' (online). Available from URL: www.nspcc.org.uk/globalassets/documents/research-reports/no-one-noticed-no-one-heard-report.pdf (accessed 28 April 2016)

Appleyard, K., Egeland, B., Van Dulmen, M. H. M. and Sroufe, L. A. (2005) 'When more is not better: The role of cumulative risk in child behavior outcomes', Journal of Child Psychology and Psychiatry, Vol. 46, No. 3, pp. 235–45; doi:10.1111/j.1469–7610.2004.00351.x

Benedict, M. I., White, R. B., Wulff, L. M. and Hall, B. J. (1990) 'Reported maltreatment in children with multiple disabilities', Child Abuse & Neglect, Vol. 14, No. 2, pp. 207–17; doi:10.1016/0145–2134(90)90031–N

Bentley, H., O'Hagan, O., Raff, A. and Bhatti, I. (2016) How safe are our children? The most comprehensive overview of child protection in the UK 2016, London: National Society for the Prevention of Cruelty to Children

Beresford, B. (ed.) (1997) Personal accounts: Involving disabled children in research, London: The Stationery Office

Bernard, C. (1999) 'Child sexual abuse and the black disabled child', Disability & Society, Vol. 14, No. 3, pp. 325–39; doi:10.1080/09687599926172

Bettenay, C., Ridley, A. M., Henry, L. A. and Crane, L. (2014), 'Cross-examination: The testimony of children with and without intellectual disabilities', Applied Cognitive Psychology, Vol. 28, No. 2, pp. 204–14; doi:10.1002/acp.2979

Boersma, J. M. F. (2008) 'Violence against Ethiopian children with disabilities: The stories and perspectives of children', Master's thesis, University of Amsterdam

Booth, T. and Booth, W. (1996) 'Sounds of silence: Narrative research with inarticulate subjects', Disability & Society, Vol. 11, No. 1, pp. 55–69; doi:10.1080/09687599650023326

Bottoms, B. L. (2003) 'Jurors' perceptions of adolescent sexual assault victims who have intellectual disabilities', Law and Human Behavior, Vol. 27, No. 2, pp. 205–27; doi:10.1023/A:1022551314668

Bradbury-Jones, C. (2014) Children as Co-Researchers: The need for protection, Protecting Children and Young People Series, Edinburgh: Dunedin Academic Press

Brandon, M., Belderson, P., Warren, C., Howe, D., Gardner, R., Dodsworth J. and Black, J. (2008) Analysing child deaths and serious injury through abuse and neglect: What can we learn? A biennial analysis of serious case reviews 2003–2005, Research Brief DCSF-RB023, London: Department for Children, Schools and Families

Brandon, M., Sidebotham, P., Bailey, S., Belderson, P., Hawley, C., Ellis, C. and Megson, M. (2012) 'New learning from serious case reviews: A two year report for 2009–2011' (online). Available from URL: www.gov.uk/government/uploads/system/uploads/attachment_data/file/184053/DFE-RR226_Report.pdf (accessed 28 April 2016)

Brennan, M. (1990) Word Formation in British Sign Language, Sweden: University of Stockholm

Broome, M. E. and Richards, D. (1998) 'Involving children in research', Journal of Child and Family Nursing, Vol. 1, No. 1, pp. 3–7

Brown, D. A. and Lewis, C. N. (2013) 'Competence is in the eye of the beholder: Perceptions of intellectually disabled child witnesses', International Journal of Disability, Development and Education, Vol. 60, No. 1, pp. 3–17; doi:10.1080/1034912X.2013.757132

Brownlie, E., Jabbar, A., Beitchman, J., Vida, R. and Atkinson, L. (2007) 'Language impairment and sexual assault of girls and women: Findings from a community sample', Journal of Abnormal Child Psychology, Vol. 35, No. 4, pp. 618–26; doi:10.1007/s10802-007-9117-4

Brownmiller, S. (1975) Against our will: Men, women, and rape, New York: Simon & Schuster

Cambridge, P. (1999) 'The first hit: A case study of the physical abuse of people with learning disabilities and challenging behaviours in a residential service', Disability & Society, Vol. 14, No. 3, pp. 285–308; doi:10.1080/09687599926154

Campbell, R. (2002) Emotionally involved: The impact of researching rape, New York: Routledge

Cavet, J. and Sloper, P. (2004) 'Participation of disabled children in individual decisions about their lives and in public decisions about service development', Children and Society, Vol. 18, No. 4, pp. 278–90; doi:10.1002/chi.803

CDC (Centers for Disease Control and Prevention) (2015) 'Short set of questions on disability. Statement of rationale for the Washington Group general measure on disability' (online). Available from URL: www.cdc.gov/nchs/data/washington_group/wg_short_measure_on_disability.pdf (accessed 15 July 2016)

Cederborg, A.-C. and Lamb, M. E. (2006) 'How does the legal system respond when children with learning difficulties are victimized?', Child Abuse & Neglect, Vol. 30, No. 5, pp. 537–47; doi:10.1016/j.chiabu.2005.10.015

Chan, K. L., Emery, C. R. and Ip, P. (2014) 'Children with disability are more at risk of violence victimization: Evidence from a study of school-aged Chinese children', Journal of Interpersonal Violence, Vol. 31, No. 6, pp. 1026–46; doi:10.1177/0886260514564066

Chapman, L. (2013) *A Different Perspective on Inclusive Practice: Respectful language. A practical handbook*, Sheffield: Centre for Welfare Reform

Christensen, P. and Prout, A. (2002) 'Working with ethical symmetry in social research with children', Childhood, Vol. 9, No. 4, pp. 477–97; doi:10.1177/0907568202009004007

Clacherty, G. and Donald, D. (2007) 'Child participation in research: Reflections on ethical challenges in the southern African context', African Journal of AIDS Research, Vol. 6, No. 2, pp. 147–56; doi:10.2989/16085900709490409

Cocks, A. (2006) 'The ethical maze: Finding an inclusive path towards gaining children's agreement to research participation', Childhood: A Global Journal of Child Research, Vol. 13, No. 2, pp. 247–66; doi:10.1177/0907568206062942

Cocks, A. (2008) 'Researching the lives of disabled children: The process of participant observation in seeking inclusivity', Qualitative Social Work, Vol. 7, No. 2, pp. 163–80; doi:10.1177/1473325008089628

Coles, J., Dartnall, E., Limjerwala, S. and Astbury, J. (2010) Researcher Trauma, Safety and Sexual Violence Research, Briefing paper, Pretoria: Sexual Violence Research Initiative

Connors, C. and Stalker, K. (2003) The Views and Experiences of Disabled Children and Their Siblings, London: Jessica Kingsley

Connors, C. and Stalker, K. (2007) 'Children's experiences of disability: Pointers to a social model of childhood disability', Disability & Society, Vol. 22, No. 1, pp. 19–33

Cooke, P. and Standen, P. J. (2002) 'Abuse and disabled children: Hidden needs…?', Child Abuse Review, Vol. 11, No. 1, pp. 1–18; doi:10.1002/car.710

CP MERG (Child Protection Monitoring and Evaluation Reference Group) (2012) Ethical principles, dilemmas and risks in collecting data on violence against children: A review of available literature, New York: UNICEF Statistics and Monitoring Section, Division of Policy and Strategy

Cree, V., Kay, H. and Tisdall, K. (2002) 'Research with children: Sharing the dilemmas', Child and Family Social Work, Vol. 7, No. 1, pp. 47–56; doi:10.1046/j.1365–2206.2002.00223.x

Crow, G., Wiles, R., Heath, S. and Charles, V. (2006) 'Research ethics and data quality: The implications of informed consent', International Journal of Social Research Methodology, Vol. 9, No. 2, pp. 83–95; doi:10.1080/13645570600595231

Devries, K. M., Kyegombe, N., Zuurmond, M., Parkes, J., Child, J. C., Walakira, E. J. and Naker, D. (2014) 'Violence against primary school children with disabilities in Uganda: A cross-sectional study', BMC Public Health, Vol. 10, No. 1; doi:10.1186/1471–2458–14–1017

Dickson-Swift, V., James, E. and Kippen, S. (2005) 'Do university ethics committees adequately protect public health researchers?', Australian and New Zealand Journal of Public Health, Vol. 29, No. 6, pp. 576–79; doi:10.1111/j.1467–842X.2005.tb00254.x

Dinos, S., Burrowes, N., Hammond, K. and Cunliffe, C. (2015) 'A systematic review of juries' assessment of rape victims: Do rape myths impact on juror decision-making?', International Journal of Law, Crime and Justice, Vol. 43, No. 1, pp. 36–49; doi:10.1016/j.ijlcj.2014.07.001

Dubowitz, H., Kim, J., Black, M. M., Weisbart, C., Semiatin, J. and Magder, L. S. (2011) 'Identifying children at high risk for a child maltreatment report', Child Abuse & Neglect, Vol. 35, No. 2, pp. 96–104; doi:10.1016/j.chiabu.2010.09.003

ESCR (Economic and Social Research Council) (n.d.) 'What is freely given informed consent' (online). Available from URL: www.esrc.ac.uk/funding/guidance-for-applicants/research-ethics/frequently-raised-questions/what-is-freely-given-informed-consent (accessed 31 January 2017)

Éthier, L. S., Lemelin, J.-P. and Lacharite, C. (2004) 'A longitudinal study of the effects of chronic maltreatment on children's behavioral and emotional problems', Child Abuse & Neglect, Vol. 28, No. 12, pp. 1265–78; doi:10.1016/j.chiabu.2004.07.006

ETHzürich (n.d.) 'z-proso – The life-course development of violence and crime' (online). Available from URL: www.cru.ethz.ch/en/projects/z-proso.html (accessed 28 June 2015)

EU FRA (European Union Agency for Fundamental Rights) (2014) 'Child participation in research' (online). Available from URL: http://fra.europa.eu/en/theme/rights-child/child-participation-in-research (accessed 19 January 2017)

Fang, X., Fry, D., Brown, D., Mercy, J., Dunne, M., Butchart, A., Corso, P., Maynzyuk, K., Dzhygyr, Y., McCoy, A. and Swales, D. (2015) 'The burden of child maltreatment in the East Asia and Pacific region', Child Abuse & Neglect, Vol. 42, pp. 146–62; doi:10.1016/j.chiabu.2015.02.012

Feldman, M., Battlin, S., Shaw, O. and Luckasson, R. (2013) 'Inclusion of children with disabilities in mainstream child development research', Disability & Society, Vol. 28, No. 7, pp. 997–1011; doi:10.1080/09687599.2012.748647

Felzmann, H., Sixsmith, J., O'Higgins, S., Ni Chonnachtaigh, S. and Nic Gabhainn, S. (2010) Ethical Review and Children's Research in Ireland, The National Children's Strategy Research Series, Dublin: Office of the Minister for Children and Youth Affairs

Finkelhor, D., Vanderminden, J., Turner, H., Hamby, S. and Shattuck, A. (2014a) 'Child maltreatment rates assessed in a national household survey of caregivers and youth', Child Abuse & Neglect, Vol. 38, No. 9, pp. 1421–35; doi:10.1016/j.chiabu.2014.05.005

Finkelhor, D., Vanderminden, J., Turner, H., Hamby, S. and Shattuck, A. (2014b) 'Upset among youth in response to questions about exposure to violence, sexual assault and family maltreatment', Child Abuse & Neglect, Vol. 38, No. 2, pp. 217–23; doi:10.1016/j.chiabu.2013.07.021

Franklin, A., Raws, P. and Smeaton, E. (2015) 'Unprotected, overprotected: Meeting the needs of young people with learning disabilities who experience, or are at risk of, sexual exploitation' (online). Available from URL: www.bild.org.uk/information/unprotected-overprotected (accessed 28 April 2016)

Fry, D. (2012) Child Maltreatment: Prevalence, incidence and consequences in the East Asia and Pacific Region, a systematic review of research, Bangkok: UNICEF East Asia and Pacific Regional Office

Fry, D., Anderson, J., Hidalgo, R. J. T., Elizalde, A., Casey, T., Rodriguez, R., Martin, A., Oroz, C., Gamarra, J., Padilla, K. and Fang, X. (2016) 'Prevalence of violence in childhood and adolescence and the impact on educational outcomes: Evidence from the 2013 Peruvian National Survey on Social Relations', International Health, Vol. 8, No. 1, pp. 44–52; doi:10.1093/inthealth/ihv075

Garcia-Moreno, C. and Watts, C. (2004) 'Doing retrospective child sexual abuse research safely and ethically with women: Is it possible?' Monash Bioethics Review, Vol. 23, No. 2, pp. S50–S59;

Garth, B. and Aroni, R. (2003) ' "I value what you have to say." Seeking the perspective of children with a disability, not just their parents', Disability & Society, Vol. 18, No. 5, pp. 561–76; doi:10.1080/0968759032000097825

Gilbert, R., Widom, C. S., Browne, K., Fergusson, D., Webb, E. and Janson, S. (2009) 'Burden and consequences of child maltreatment in high-income countries', The Lancet, Vol. 373, No. 9657, pp. 68–81; doi:10.1016/S0140-6736(08)61706-7

Gilligan, R. (2015) 'Children's rights and disability', in Iriarte, E. G., McConkey, R. and Gilligan, R. (eds) (2015). Disability and Human Rights: Global Perspectives, London: Palgrave Macmillan

Gorin, S., Hooper, C. A., Dyson, C. and Cabral, C. (2008) 'Ethical challenges in conducting research with hard to reach families', Child Abuse Review, Vol. 17, No. 4, pp. 275–87; doi:10.1002/car.1031

Graham, A., Powell, M., Taylor, N., Anderson, D. and Fitzgerald, R. (2013) Ethical Research Involving Children, Florence: UNICEF Office of Research–Innocenti

Groce, N. (2005) Violence against children with disabilities: UN Secretary General's study on violence against children thematic group on violence against children with disabilities, New York: UNICEF

Harrell, E. (2012) 'Crime against persons with disabilities, 2009–11: Statistical tables' (online). Available from URL: www.bjs.gov/index.cfm?ty=pbdetail&iid=4574 (accessed 28 April 2016)

Helton, J. J. and Bruhn, C. M. (2013) 'Prevalence of disabilities and abilities in children investigated for abuse and neglect', Journal of Public Child Welfare, Vol. 7, No. 5, pp. 480–95; doi:10.1080/15548732.2013.843497

Helton, J. J. and Cross, T. P. (2011) 'The relationship of child functioning to parental physical assault: Linear and curvilinear models', Child Maltreatment, Vol. 16, No. 2, pp. 126–36; doi:10.1177/1077559511401742.

Henry, L., Ridley, A., Perry, J. and Crane, L. (2011) 'Perceived credibility and eyewitness testimony of children with intellectual disabilities', Journal of Intellectual Disability Research, Vol. 55, No. 4, pp. 385–91; doi:10.1111/j.1365-2788.2011.01383.x

Hershkowitz, I., Lamb, M. E. and Horowitz, D. (2007) 'Victimization of children with disabilities', American Journal of Orthopsychiatry, Vol. 77, No. 4, pp. 629–35; doi:10.1037/0002-9432.77.4.629

Hibbard, R. A., Desch, L. W. and the Committee on Child Abuse and Neglect and Council on Children With Disabilities (2007) 'Maltreatment of children with disabilities', Pediatrics, Vol. 119, No. 5, pp. 1018–25; doi:10.1542/peds.2007–0565

Hildyard, K. L. and Wolfe, D. A. (2002) 'Child neglect: Developmental issues and outcomes', Child Abuse & Neglect, Vol. 26, Nos 6–7, pp. 679–95; doi:10.1016/S0145-2134(02)00341-1

Hillis, S., Mercy, J., Saul, J., Gleckel, J., Abad, N. and Kress, H. (2015) THRIVES: A global package to prevent violence against children, Atlanta, GA: Centers for Disease Control and Prevention

Hillis, S., Mercy, J., Amobi, A. and Kress, H. (2016) 'Global prevalence of past-year violence against children: A systematic review and minimum estimates', Pediatrics, Vol. 137, No. 3, pp. 1–13; doi:e20154079

Hulipas, E. J. (2005) 'The inner world of the sexually abused adolescents with mental retardation at the National Center for Mental Health–Women and Children Protection Unit' (online). Available from URL: www.elib.gov.ph/details.php?uid=7d1bff4a8d183a665d34e5f6197041ee&tab=2 (accessed 19 January 2017)

Hunter, D. and Pierscionek, B. (2007) 'Children, Gillick competency and consent for involvement in research', Journal of Medical Ethics, Vol. 33, No. 11, pp. 659–62; doi:10.1136/jme.2006.018853

IDDC (International Disability and Development Consortium) (2016) 'The 2030 agenda: The inclusion of persons with disabilities' (online). Available from URL: www.iddcconsortium.net/resources-tools/2030-agenda-inclusion-persons-disabilities (accessed 16 February 2017)

ISPCAN (International Society for the Prevention of Child Abuse and Neglect) (2016) Ethical Considerations for the Collection, Analysis & Publication of Child Maltreatment Data, Chicago, IL: ISPCAN

Jones, A. (2004) 'Involving children and young people as researchers', in Fraser, S., Lewis, V., Ding, S., Kellett, M. and Robinson, C. (eds) (2004) Doing Research with Children and Young People, London: Sage

Jones, C., Stalker, K., Franklin, A., Fry, D., Cameron, A. and Taylor, J. (2016) 'Enablers of help-seeking for deaf and disabled children following abuse and barriers to protection: A qualitative study', Child and Family Social Work; doi:10.1111/cfs.12293

Jones, L., Bellis, M. A., Wood, S., Hughes, K., McCoy, E., Eckley, L., Bates, G., Mikton, C., Shakespeare, T. and Officer, A. (2012) 'Prevalence and risk of violence against children with disabilities: A systematic review and meta-analysis of observational studies', The Lancet, Vol. 380, No. 9845, pp. 899–907; doi:10.1016/S0140-6736(12)60692-8

Katz, J. (1996) 'The Nuremberg code and the Nuremberg trial: A reappraisal', Journal of the American Medical Association, Vol. 276, No. 20, pp. 1662–6

Kelly, B. (2007) 'Methodological issues for qualitative research with learning disabled children', International Journal of Social Research Methodology, Vol. 10, No. 1, pp. 21–35; doi:10.1080/13645570600655159

Kelly, B. and Dowling, S. (2015) Safeguarding Disabled Children and Young People: A scoping exercise of statutory child protection services for disabled children and young people in Northern Ireland, Belfast: Queen's University and Safeguarding Board for Northern Ireland

Kelly, B., Dowling, S. and Winter, K. (2016) Addressing the Needs and Experiences of Disabled Children and Young People in Out-Of-Home Care, Belfast: Queen's University and Office of First Minister & Deputy First Minister

Kendall-Tackett, K., Lyon, T., Talieferro, G. and Little, L. (2005) 'Why child maltreatment researchers should include children's disability status in their maltreatment studies', Child Abuse & Neglect, Vol. 29, No. 2, pp. 147–51; doi:10.1016/j.chiabu.2004.09.002

Knight, E. D., Runyan, D. K., Dubowitz, H., Brandford, C., Kotch, J., Litrownik, A. and Hunter, W. (2000) 'Methodological and ethical challenges associated with child self-report of maltreatment solutions implemented by the LONGSCAN consortium', Journal of Interpersonal Violence, Vol. 15, No. 7, pp. 760–75; doi:10.1177/088626000015007006

Knox, M., Mok, M. and Parmenter, T. (2000) 'Working with the experts: Collaborative research with people with an intellectual disability', Disability & Society, Vol. 15, No. 1, pp. 49–61

Koetting, C., Fitzpatrick, J. J., Lewin, L. and Kilanowski, J. (2012) 'Nurse practitioner knowledge of child sexual abuse in children with cognitive disabilities', Journal of Forensic Nursing, Vol. 8, No. 2, pp. 72–80; doi:10.1111/j.1939-3938.2011.01129.x

Krug, E. G., Dahlberg, L. L., Mercy, J. A., Zwi, A. B. and Lozano, R. (eds) (2002) World Report on Violence and Health, Geneva: World Health Organization

Krüger, P., Schmitz, S. C. and Niehaus, S. (2014) 'Mythen geistiger Behinderung und sexueller Gewalt im Strafverfahren', Vierteljahresschrift für Heilpädagogik und ihre Nachbargebiete, Vol. 83, No. 2, pp. 124–36; doi:10.2378/vhn2013.art

Kuper, H., Banks, M., Kelly, S., Kyegombe, N. and Devries, K. (2016) Protect Us! Inclusion of children with disabilities in child protection, Woking: Plan International

Kvam, M. H. (2000) 'Is sexual abuse of children with disabilities disclosed? A retrospective analysis of child disability and the likelihood of sexual abuse among those attending Norwegian hospitals', Child Abuse & Neglect, Vol. 24, No. 8, pp. 1073–84; doi:10.1016/S0145-2134(00)00159-9

Kvam, M. H. (2004) 'Sexual abuse of deaf children. A retrospective analysis of the prevalence and characteristics of childhood sexual abuse among deaf adults in Norway', Child Abuse & Neglect, Vol. 28, No. 3, pp. 241–51; doi:10.1016/j.chiabu.2003.09.017

Lamprecht, L. (2003) 'Sexuality in children with intellectual disabilities', presented at a workshop of the South African Association for Scientific Study of Mental Handicap, Johannesburg general hospital

Lee, J.-S., Bartolomei, L. and Pittaway, E. (2016) 'Survey research with preliterate adult populations in post conflict situations using researcher-assisted self-completion questionnaires', International Journal of Social Research Methodology, Vol. 19, No. 6, pp. 717–30; doi:10.1080/13645579.2015.1091236

Leeb, R. T., Bitsko, R. H., Merrick, M. T. and Armour, B. S. (2012) 'Does childhood disability increase risk for child abuse and neglect?', Journal of Mental Health Research in Intellectual Disabilities, Vol. 5, No. 1, pp. 4–31; doi:10.1080/19315864.2011.608154

Levine, R. J. (1988) Ethics and Regulations of Clinical Research, New Haven, CT: Yale University Press

Lewis, A. and Porter, J. (2004) 'Interviewing children and young people with learning disabilities: Guidelines for researchers and multi-professional practice', British Journal of Learning Disabilities, Vol. 32, No. 4, pp. 191–7; doi:10.1111/j.1468-3156.2004.00313.x

Lightfoot, E. B. and LaLiberte, T. L. (2006) 'Approaches to child protection case management for cases involving people with disabilities', Child Abuse & Neglect, Vol. 30, No. 4, pp. 381–91; doi:10.1016/j.chiabu.2005.10.013

Lightfoot, E., Hill, K. and LaLiberte, T. (2011) 'Prevalence of children with disabilities in the child welfare system and out of home placement: An examination of administrative records', Children and Youth Services Review, Vol. 33, No. 11, pp. 2069–75; doi:10.1016/j.childyouth.2011.02.019

Lonsway, K. A. and Fitzgerald, L. F. (1994) 'Rape myths in review', Psychology of Women Quarterly, Vol. 18, No. 2, pp. 133–64; doi:10.1111/j.1471–6402.1994.tb00448.x

Loveridge, J. and Meyer, L. (2010) 'Involving children and young people in research in educational settings' (online). Available from URL: www.education-counts.govt.nz/publications/schooling/80440/Chapter_1 (accessed 27 April 2016)

Macarthur, J., Gaffney, M., Sharp, S. and Kelly, B. (2007) 'Disabled children negotiating school life: Agency, difference and teaching practice', The International Journal of Children's Rights, Vol. 15, No. 1, pp. 99–120; doi:10.1163/092755607X181720

McCarthy, M. and Thompson, D. (1996) 'Sexual abuse by design: An examination of the issues in learning disability services', Disability & Society, Vol. 11, No. 2, pp. 205–18; doi:10.1080/09687599650023236

McElvaney, R., Greene, S. and Hogan, D. (2014) 'To tell or not to tell? Factors influencing young people's informal disclosures of child sexual abuse', Journal of Interpersonal Violence, Vol. 29, No. 928; doi:10.1177/0886260513506281

McKee, M., Schlehofer, D. and Thew, D. (2013) 'Ethical issues in conduction research with deaf populations', American Journal of Public Health, Vol. 103, No. 12, pp. 2174–8; doi:10.2105/AJPH.2013.301343

Maier, T., Mohler-Kuo, M., Landolt, M. A., Schnyder, U. and Jud, A. (2013) 'The tip of the iceberg. Incidence of disclosed cases of child sexual abuse in Switzerland: Results from a nationwide agency survey', International Journal of Public Health, Vol. 58, No. 6, pp. 875–83; doi:10.1007/s00038–013–0498–6

Mallen, A. (2011) ' "It's like piecing together small pieces of a puzzle": Difficulties in reporting abuse and neglect of disabled children to the social services', Journal of Scandinavian Studies in Criminology and Crime Prevention, Vol. 12, pp. 45–62

Manders, J. E. and Stoneman, Z. (2009) 'Children with disabilities in the child protective services system: An analog study of investigation and case management', Child Abuse & Neglect, Vol. 33, No. 4, pp. 229–37; doi:10.1016/j.chiabu.2008.10.001

Manly, J. T., Kim, J. E., Rogosch, F. A. and Cicchetti, D. (2001) 'Dimensions of child maltreatment and children's adjustment: Contributions of developmental timing and subtype', Development and Psychopathology, Vol. 13, No. 4, pp. 759–82

Margolin, G. and Gordis, E. B. (2004) 'Children's exposure to violence in the family and community', Current Directions in Psychological Science, Vol. 13, No. 4, pp. 152–5; doi:10.1111/j.0963–7214.2004.00296.x

Mikkelson, H. (2000) 'Interpreter ethics: A review of the traditional and electronic literature', Interpreting, Vol. 5, No. 1, pp. 49–56; doi:10.1075/intp.5.1.05mik

Miller, T. and Boulton, M. (2007) 'Changing constructions of informed consent: Qualitative research and complex social worlds', Social Science and Medicine, Vol. 65, No. 11, pp. 2199–211; doi:10.1016/j.socscimed.2007.08.009

Mitchell, W. and Sloper, P. (2011) 'Making choices in my life: Listening to the ideas and experiences of young people in the UK who communicate non-verbally', Children and Youth Services Review, Vol. 33, No. 4, pp. 521–7; doi:10.1016/j.childyouth.2010.05.016

Morris, A., Hegarty, K. and Humphreys, C. (2012) 'Ethical and safe: Research with children about domestic violence', Research Ethics, Vol. 8, No. 2, pp. 125–39; doi:10.1177/1747016112445420

Morrow, V. (2011) Understanding Children and Childhood, Background Briefing Series No. 1, Lismore, Australia: Centre for Children and Young People, Southern Cross University

Munro, E. (2011). The Munro Review of Child Protection: Part one: A systems analysis, London: Department for Education

Napier, J., McKee, R. L. and Goswell, D. (2010) Sign Language Interpreting (2nd edn), Sydney: The Federation Press

NIDCD (National institute on deafness and other communication disorders) (1999) 'Working Group on Communicating Informed Consent to Individuals Who Are Deaf or Hard-of-Hearing' (online). Available from URL: www.nidcd. nih.gov/workshops/communicating-informed-consent-individuals-who-are-deaf-hard-of-hearing/1999 (accessed 27 April 2016)

Niehaus, S., Krüger, P. and Schmitz, S. C. (2013) 'Intellectually disabled victims of sexual abuse in the criminal justice system', Psychology, Vol. 4, No. 3, pp. 374–9; doi:10.4236/psych.2013.43A054

Nind, M. (2008) 'Conducting qualitative research with people with learning, communication and other disabilities: Methodological challenges' (online). Available from URL: http://eprints.ncrm.ac.uk/491 (accessed 28 April 2016)

Nowak, C. B. (2015) 'Recognition and prevention of child abuse in the child with disability', American Journal of Medical Genetics Part C: Seminars in Medical Genetics, Vol. 169, No. 4, pp. 293–301; doi:10.1002/ajmg.c.31458

Odell, T. (2011) 'Not your average childhood: Lived experience of children with physical disabilities raised in Bloorview Hospital, Home and School from 1960 to 1989', Disability & Society, Vol. 26, No. 1, pp. 49–63; doi:10.1080/0968759 9.2011.529666

Oosterhoorn, R. and Kendrick, A. (2001) 'No sign of harm: Issues for disabled children communicating about abuse', Child Abuse Review, Vol. 10, No. 4, pp. 243–53; doi:10.1002/car.697

Orelove, F. P., Hollahan, D. J. and Myles, K. T. (2000) 'Maltreatment of children with disabilities: Training needs for a collaborative response', Child Abuse & Neglect, Vol. 24, No. 2, pp. 185–94; doi:10.1016/S0145–2134(99)00134–9

Ouyang, L., Fang, X., Mercy, J., Perou, R. and Grosse, S. D. (2008) 'Attention-deficit/hyperactivity disorder symptoms and child maltreatment: A population-based study', The Journal of Pediatrics, Vol. 153, No. 6, pp. 851–56; doi:10.1016/j.jpeds.2008.06.002

Palmer, M. and Harley, D. (2012) 'Models and measurement in disability: An international review', Health Policy and Planning, Vol. 27, No. 5, pp. 357–64; doi:10.1093/heapol/czr047

Parsons, S., Sherwood, G. and Abbott, C. (2016) 'Informed consent with children and young people in social research: Is there scope for innovation?', Children and Society, Vol. 30, No. 2, pp. 132–45; doi:10.1111/chso.12117

Pearlman, L. and Saakvitne, K. (eds). (1995). Trauma and the Therapist: Countertransference and vicarious traumatization in psychotherapy with incest survivors, New York, NY: Norton

Pereda, N., Guilera, G., Forns, M. and Gómez-Benito, J. (2009) 'The international epidemiology of child sexual abuse: A continuation of Finkelhor (1994)', Child Abuse & Neglect, Vol. 33, No. 6, pp. 331–42; doi:10.1016/j.chiabu.2008.07.007

Petersilia, J. R. (2001) 'Crime victims with developmental disabilities', Criminal Justice and Behavior, Vol. 28, No. 6, pp. 655–94; doi:10.1177/009385480102800601

Pfeffer, R. (2014) 'Risk and protective factors for the safety of children with autism: A qualitative study of caregivers' perspectives', Journal of Family Strengths, Vol. 14, No. 1, Art. 21. Available from URL:

Pinheiro, P. S. (2006) 'World report on violence against children: United Nations Secretary-General's study on violence against children' (online). Available from URL: www.unicef.org/violencestudy/reports/SG_violencestudy_en.pdf (accessed 28 April 2016)

Pittaway, E, Bartolomei, L. and Lee, J. S. (in prep.) Evaluating Anti-Oppressive Practice with Sexually Abused Disabled Children and Their Families in Burundi (working title)

Pollard, R. Q. Jr, Dean, R. K., O'Hearn, A. and Haynes, S. L. (2009) 'Adapting health education material for Deaf audiences', Rehabilitation Psychology, Vol. 54, No. 2, pp. 232–8; doi:10.1037/a0015772

Pollard, R. Q. Jr, Betts, W. R., Carroll, J. K., Waxmonsky, J. A., Barnett, S., deGruy, F. V. III, Pickler, L. and Kellar-Guenther, Y. (2014) 'Integrating primary care and behavioural health with four special populations: Children with special needs, people with serious mental illness, refugees and deaf people', American Psychologist, Vol. 69, No. 4, pp. 377–97; doi:10.1037/a0036220

Public Health Agency of Canada (2010) Canadian Incidence Study of Reported Child Abuse and Neglect – 2008: Major Findings, Ottawa: Public Health Agency of Canada. Available from URL: http://cwrp.ca/sites/default/files/publications/en/CIS-2008-rprt-eng.pdf (accessed 26 August 2015)

Rabiee, P., Sloper, P. and Beresford, B. (2005) 'Doing research with children and young people who do not use speech for communication', Children and Society, Vol. 19, No. 5, pp. 385–96; doi:10.1002/chi.841

Radford, L., Corral, S., Bradely, C., Fisher, H., Bassett, C., Howat, N. and Collishaw, S. (2011) Child Abuse and Neglect in the UK Today, London: National Society for the Prevention of Cruelty to Children

Ranalidi, F. and Nisbet, P. (2010) A Teacher's Guide to Creating Accessible Learning Resources, Edinburgh: CALL Scotland, University of Edinburgh

Reiman, E. (2014) 'Implicit bias about disabilities: Does it exist for forensic interviewers and could it affect child credibility decisions in child abuse investigations: An exploratory study' (online). Available from URL: http://

academicworks.cuny.edu/cgi/viewcontent.cgi?article=1465&context=gc_etds (accessed 7 March 2016)

Reiter, S., Bryen, D. N. and Shachar, I. (2007) 'Adolescents with intellectual disabilities as victims of abuse', Journal of Intellectual Disabilities, Vol. 11, No. 4, pp. 371–87; doi:10.1177/1744629507084602

RNIB (Royal National Institute of the Blind) (n.d.) 'What font size is large print?' (online). Available from URL: https://help.rnib.org.uk/help/daily-living/reading/large-print-size (accessed 27 April 2016)

Roberts, G., Anderson, P. J., Doyle, L. W. and Victorian Infant Collaborative Study Group (2010) 'The stability of the diagnosis of developmental disability between ages 2 and 8 in a geographic cohort of very preterm children born in 1997', Archives of disease in childhood, Vol. 95, No. 10, pp. 786–90; doi:10.1136/adc.2009.160283

Rodgers, J. (1999) 'Trying to get it right: Undertaking research involving people with learning difficulties', Disability & Society, Vol. 14, No. 4, pp. 421–33

Rodriguez, E. S. and Guerrero, A. R. (2002) 'An international perspective: What are ethics for sign language interpreters? A comparative study among different codes of ethics', Journal of Interpretation, pp. 49–61

Rogers, P., Titterington, L. and Davies, M. (2009) 'Attributions of blame and credibility in a hypothetical child sexual abuse case: Roles of victim disability, victim resistance and respondent gender', International Journal of Disability, Development and Education, Vol. 56, No. 3, pp. 205–28; doi:10.1080/10349120903102189

Roy, C. B. (ed.) (2000) Innovative Practices for Teaching Sign Language Interpreters, Washington, DC: Gallaudet University Press

SACG (South Asia Coordinating Group on Action against Violence against Children) and SAIEVAC (South Asia Initiative to End Violence Against Children) (2016) Implementation of the Sustainable Development Goals Relating to Violence against Children in South Asia: Background document, Colombo, Sri Lanka: SAIEVAC

SAIEVAC (South Asia Initiative to End Violence Against Children) (2014) 'Report of the 4th technical consultation on stepping up protection of children with disabilities in South Asia. 3–7 December 2014 in Sri Lanka' (online). Available from URL: www.civilsocietyasia.org/uploads/resources/53/attachment/Report%20-%204th%20Technical%20Consultation%20(RS).pdf (accessed 9 February 2017)

Save the Children and Handicap International (2011) Out from the Shadows: Sexual violence against children with disabilities, London: Save the Children

Schwendinger, J. R. and Schwendinger, H. (1974) 'Rape myths: In legal, theoretical, and everyday practice', Crime and Social Justice, Vol. 1, pp. 18–26

Sedlak, A. J., Mettenburg, J., Basena, M., Petta, L., McPherson, K., Greene, A. and Li, S. (2010) Fourth National Incidence Study of Child Abuse and Neglect (NIS-4): Report to Congress, Washington, DC, US Department of Health and Human Services, Administration for Children and Families. Available from URL: www.acf.hhs.gov/sites/default/files/opre/nis4_report_congress_full_pdf_jan2010.pdf (accessed 28 April 2016)

Senn, C. Y. (1988) Vulnerable: Sexual abuse and people with an intellectual handicap, Toronto: The G. Allan Roeher Institute; doi:10.1002/car.2380010316

Shannon, P. and Tappan, C. (2011) 'Identification and assessment of children with developmental disabilities in child welfare' Social Work, Vol. 56, No. 4, pp. 297–305; doi:10.1093/sw/56.4.297

Singleton, J., Jones, G. and Hanumantha, S. (2014) 'Toward ethical research practice with Deaf participants', Journal of Empirical Research on Human Research Ethics, Vol. 9, No. 3, pp. 59–66; doi:10.1177/1556264614540589

Spencer, N., Devereux, E., Wallace, A., Sundrum, R., Shenoy, M., Bacchus, C. and Logan, S. (2005) 'Disabling conditions and registration for child abuse and neglect: A population-based study', Pediatrics, Vol. 116, No. 3, pp. 609–13; doi:10.1542/peds.2004–1882

Sprang, G., Clark, J. J. and Bass, S. (2005) 'Factors that contribute to child maltreatment severity: A multi-method and multidimensional investigation', Child Abuse & Neglect, Vol. 29, No. 4, pp. 335–50; doi:10.1016/j.chiabu.2004.08.008

Stalker, K. (2013) 'Safeguarding deaf and disabled children: A resource for use in training and professional group learning', Child Abuse Review, Vol. 22, No. 2, pp. 142–5; doi:10.1002/car.2210

Stalker, K. and McArthur, K. (2012) 'Child abuse, child protection and disabled children: A review of recent research', Child Abuse Review, Vol. 21, No. 1, pp. 24–40; doi:10.1002/car.1154

Stalker, K., Green Lister, P., Lerpiniere, J. and McArthur, K. (2010) Child Protection and the Needs and Rights of Disabled Children and Young People: A scoping study, Glasgow: University of Strathclyde

Stalker, K., Taylor, J., Fry, D. and Stewart, A. B. R. (2015) 'A study of disabled children and child protection in Scotland – A hidden group?', Children and Youth Services Review, Vol. 56, pp. 126–34; doi:10.1016/j.childyouth.2015.07.012

Stoltenborgh, M., van Ijzendoorn, M. H., Euser, E. M. and Bakermans-Kranenburg, M. J. (2011) 'A global perspective on child sexual abuse: Meta-analysis of prevalence around the world', Child Maltreatment, Vol. 16, No. 2, pp. 79–101; doi:10.1177/1077559511403920

Stoltenborgh, M., Bakermans–Kranenburg, M. J., Alink, L. R. A. and Van Ijzendoorn, M. H. (2012) 'The universality of childhood emotional abuse: A meta-analysis of worldwide prevalence.' Journal of Aggression, Maltreatment & Trauma, Vol. 21, pp. 870–90; doi:10.1080/10926771.2012.708014

Stoltenborgh, M., Bakermans-Kranenburg, M. J., Van Ijzendoorn, M. H. and Alink, L. R. A. (2013) 'Cultural–geographical differences in the occurrence of child physical abuse? A meta-analysis of global prevalence', International Journal of Psychology, Vol. 48, No. 2, pp. 81–94; doi:10.1080/00207594.2012.697165

Stöpler, L. (2007) Hidden Shame: Violence against children with disabilities in East Africa, Den Haag: Terre des Hommes Netherland

Sudore, R., Landefeld, S., Williams, B., Barnes, D., Lindquits, K. and Schillinger, D. (2006) 'Use of a modified informed consent process among vulnerable patients: A descriptive study', Journal of General Internal Medicine, Vol. 21, No. 8, pp. 867–73; doi:10.1111/j.1525–1497.2006.00535.x

Sullivan, P. M. (2009) 'Violence exposure among children with disabilities', Clinical Child and Family Psychology Review, Vol. 12, No. 2, pp. 196–216; doi:10.1007/s10567–009–0056–1.

Sullivan, P. M. and Knutson, J. F. (2000) 'Maltreatment and disabilities: A population-based epidemiological study', Child Abuse & Neglect, Vol. 24, No. 10, pp. 1257–73; doi:10.1016/S0145-2134(00)00190-3

Sutton-Spence, R. and Woll, B. (1999) The Linguistics of British Sign Language: An introduction, Cambridge: Cambridge University Press

Tarleton, B., Williams, V., Palmer, N. and Gramlich, S. (2004) 'An equal relationship?: People with learning difficulties getting involved with research', in Smyth, M. and Williamson, W. (eds) (2004) Researchers and Their 'Subjects': Ethics, power, knowledge and consent, Bristol: Policy Press, pp. 73–88

Taylor, J., Stalker, K., Fry, D. and Stewart, A. (2014) Disabled Children and Child Protection in Scotland: An investigation into the relationship between professional practice, child protection and disability, Research Findings No. 127/2014, Edinburgh: Scottish Government Children's Rights and Wellbeing Division

Taylor, J., Cameron, A., Jones, C., Franklin, A., Stalker, K. and Fry, D. (2015a) Deaf and Disabled Children Talking about Child Protection, Edinburgh: The University of Edinburgh/NSPCC Child Protection Research Centre

Taylor, J., Stalker, K. and Stewart, A. (2015b) 'Disabled children and the child protection system: A cause for concern', Child Abuse Review, Vol. 25, No. 1, pp. 60–73; doi:10.1002/car.2386

Terol, E. H. (2009) 'Cases of sexually abused adolescent girls with mental retardation in the Philippines', Journal of Child and Adolescent Trauma, Vol. 2, No. 3, pp. 209–27; doi:10.1080/19361520903120525

Thompson, R., Zuroff, D. C. and Hindi, E. (2012) 'Relationships and traumatic events as predictors of depressive styles in high-risk youth', Personality and Individual Differences, Vol. 53, No. 4, pp. 474–9; doi:10.1016/j.paid.2012.04.017

Tiwari, A., Fong, D. Y. T., Chan, K. L., Leung, W. C., Parker, B. and Ho, P. C. (2007) 'Identifying intimate partner violence: Comparing the Chinese abuse assessment screen with the Chinese revised conflict tactics scales', BJOG: An International Journal of Obstetrics & Gynaecology, Vol. 114, No. 9, pp. 1065–71; doi:10.1111/j.1471-0528.2007.01441.x

Tremblay, R. E., Vitaro, F., Gagnon, C., Piché, C. and Royer, N. (1992) 'A prosocial scale for the preschool behaviour questionnaire: Concurrent and predictive correlates', International Journal of Behavioral Development, Vol. 15, No. 2, pp. 227–45; doi:10.1177/016502549201500204

Trickett, P. K. and McBride-Chang, C. (1995) 'The developmental impact of different forms of child abuse and neglect', Developmental Review, Vol. 15, No. 3, pp. 311–37; doi:10.1006/drev.1995.1012

Turner, H. A., Finkelhor, D. and Ormrod, R. (2009) 'Child mental health problems as risk factors for victimization', Child Maltreatment, Vol. 15, No. 2, pp. 132–43; doi:10.1177/1077559509349450

Turner, H. A., Vanderminden, J., Finkelhor, D., Hamby, S. and Shattuck, A. (2011) 'Disability and victimization in a national sample of children and youth', Child Maltreatment, Vol. 16, No. 4, pp. 275–86; doi:10.1177/1077559511427178.

UNICEF (United Nations Children's Fund) (2005) 'Summary report: Violence against disabled children; Findings and recommendations of a consultation convened by UNICEF New York, 28 July 2005 for the UN Secretary General's study on violence against children, thematic group on violence against children with disabilities' (online). Available from URL: www.unicef.org/videoaudio/PDFs/UNICEF_Violence_Against_Disabled_Children_Report_Distributed_Version.pdf (accessed 9 February 2017)

UNICEF (2012) Measuring and Monitoring Child Protection Systems: Proposed core indicators for the East Asia and Pacific Region, Strengthening Child Protection Series No. 1, Bangkok: UNICEF East Asia and the Pacific Regional Office

UNICEF (2013) The State of the World's Children: Children with disabilities, New York: UNICEF

United Nations Committee on the Rights of the Child (2007) 'General Comment No. 9, the rights of children with disabilities', UN document crc/c/gc/9, February

United Nations General Assembly (1989) Convention on the Rights of the Child, Geneva: United Nations

United Nations General Assembly (2006) Convention on the Rights of People with Disabilities, New York, NY: United Nations

United Nations General Assembly (2014) Fundamental Principles of Official Statistics, Resolution 68/261, New York, NY: United Nations

United Nations General Assembly (2015) *Transforming Our World: The 2030 agenda for sustainable development*, A/RES/70/1, New York, NY: United Nations

University of Sheffield (2015) 'Specialist guidance on ethical issues: Doing research with people with learning disabilities' (online). Available from URL: www.sheffield.ac.uk/ris/other/gov-ethics/ethicspolicy/further-guidance/special-guidance (accessed 19 January 2017)

UPIAS (Union of the Physically Impaired Against Segregation) (1975) 'Fundamental Principles' (online). Available from URL: www.leeds.ac.uk/disability-studies/archiveuk/archframe.htm

Ward, L. (1997) Seen and Heard: Involving disabled children and young people in research and development projects, York: Joseph Rowntree Foundation

Weindling, P. (2001) 'The origins of informed consent: The international scientific commission on medical war crimes, and the Nuremberg Code', Bulletin of the History of Medicine, Vol. 75, No. 1, pp. 37–71

Westcott, H. L. and Jones, D. P. H. (1999) 'Annotation: The abuse of disabled children', Journal of Child Psychology and Psychiatry, Vol. 40, No. 4, pp. 497–506; doi:10.1111/1469-7610.00468

WHO (2007) WHO Ethical and Safety Recommendations for Researching, Documenting and Monitoring Sexual Violence in Emergencies, Geneva: World Health Organization

WHO and World Bank (2011) World Report on Disability, Geneva: World Health Organization

Wilczynski, S. M., Connolly, S., Dubard, M., Henderson, A. and McIntosh, D. (2015) 'Assessment, prevention, and intervention for abuse among individuals with disabilities', Psychology in the Schools, Vol. 52, No. 1, pp. 9–21; doi:10.1002/pits.21808

Wiles, R., Crow, G., Charles, V. and Heath, S. (2007) 'Informed consent and the research process: Following rules or striking balances?', Sociological Research Online, Vol. 12, No. 2; doi:10.5153/sro.1208

Wilson, E., Pollock, K. and Aubeeluck, A. (2010) 'Gaining and maintaining consent when capacity can be an issue: A research study with people with Huntington's disease', Clinical Ethics, Vol. 5, pp. 142–7

Woodward, J. (1972) 'Implications for sociolinguistic research among the deaf', Sign Language Studies, Vol. 1, pp. 1–7; doi:10.1353/sls/1972.0004

Yoon, S. J. (2016) 'Ethical considerations in research with children: Focusing on children's right to participation', Journal for Korean Council for Children & Rights, Vol. 20, No. 2

Young, A. and Hunt. R. (2011) 'Research with d/Deaf people' (online). Available from URL: www.lse.ac.uk/LSEHealthAndSocialCare/pdf/SSCR%20 Methods%20Review_9_web.pdf (accessed 27 April 2016)

Young, A. and Temple, B. (2014) Approaches to Social Research: The case of Deaf studies, New York< NY: Oxford University Press

Zimmerman, C. and Watts, C. (2003) WHO Ethical and Safety Recommendations for Interviewing Trafficked Women, Geneva: World Health Organization

INDEX

Note: page numbers in italics refer to figures